Intermittent Fasting

*The Complete Guide For Weight Loss,
Burn Fat Through Meal Plan, Healing
your Body for a Healthy Lifestyle.*

Table of Contents

Disclaimer:

Introduction

Congratulations on downloading *"Intermittent Fasting: The Complete Guide For Weight Loss, Burn Fat Through Meal Plan, Healing your Body for a Healthy Lifestyle."* and thank you for doing so.

There is something that must have sparked your interest in intermittent fasting, and I hope that I can give insight into why intermittent fasting is a lifestyle that anyone can and should do.

There are lots of people who struggle with their weight. They jump back and forth between fad diet after fad diet, only to see limited to no results. Some people may go to the gym one week and refuse to do so right after. They have no motivation or desire to be healthy. Other people are so busy with their families and careers that they do not have time to give attention to their health, especially their diet. These people pick up fast food on the way to work and back home, taking a significant hit on their bodies in the process. Other people are interested in being healthy but have no idea where to begin.

Everyone knows that you should prioritize your health, but if you have never been talked or seen healthy habits practiced, they run around like a chicken with its head cut off. Feeling discouraged about not knowing where to begin their health (if they even care at all), these people just give up and succumb to a lifestyle of unhealthy eating and habits. All of us have been one of these people in life. Maybe you are one of these people who has hit rock bottom, and you know that you have to do something about your health or you will suffer dire consequences. Look no further for the solution you are looking for because it is all in this book.

There is a way for you to get your weight under control and to be the healthy person that you know you can be. This method also works for people who are already healthy. The easiest way to get healthy is to gain control of your diet. If you can control your diet, gaining or losing weight becomes a lot easier. Even for those who have had a struggle with their diet, there is still help. The easiest way to get your diet under control is by intermittent fasting. Intermittent fasting is all about limiting the time that you eat, with a focus on eating healthy foods every eating time. Ultimately, intermittent fasting helps maintain your healthy portion control and lends itself to an overall improvement in one's health. It enables you to fight sugar cravings and unsavory inflammatory illnesses that can hinder one for life.

Intermittent fasting is easy, simple, and a relatively painless way to lead a healthier lifestyle. Once you understand its basic principles, you can find ways to incorporate the changes within your lifestyle for maximum health gains. With this book, there are no more excuses that will hinder you from committing to this lifestyle. Everything you need to begin and sustain intermittent fasting is laid out for you plain and simple in this book. This book is grateful to be a part of your transformation and commitment to a healthier lifestyle. Thank you for making a commitment to yourself and to the people who care about you. By the time you finish reading, you'll be able to discuss intermittent fasting with ease and conviction as a proud practitioner.

The following chapters will discuss everything you need to know about fasting. Chapter One explores what fasting is and why it is right for you. Chapter Two explains how to fast. Different fasting methods are discussed in the Third Chapter, and Chapter Four gives fasting tips and answers to frequently asked questions about fasting. Chapter Five, meanwhile, gives you a few easy recipes that will help you start your fasting journey. Be sure to take notes about every information you find appealing. It will help you find it easier for future reference.

Before you start going through the pages, I say, "Happy reading!" And by the time you finish, I hope I can say, "Happy Fasting!"

There are plenty of books on this subject on the market, thanks again for choosing this one! Every effort was made to ensure it is full of as much useful information as possible. Please enjoy!

Chapter 1: What is Fasting and Why it is Good for You?

Why would one be interested in fasting? Why would someone forego their favorite foods to get healthier? This chapter will explain everything fasting and show you the advantages fasting can have in your life. Fasting has been important to many cultures all around the world. This chapter will give a brief overview of what fasting is, a short history, and end with the many benefits it has for people who want to lose weight, control type 2 diabetes, look younger, and improve their heart health. The chapter will end with a word of caution and give groups of people who should probably avoid fasting.

Fasting and starvation are often lumped together, but they are different. When a person starves, they do not have any food to eat, whereas, fasting is the purposeful foregoing of food. Starvation is out of a person's control; fasting is done by a person in control. Lots of people reported mental clarity, a decrease in digestion issues, weight loss, easier sleeping, and a simpler, cleaner, more convenient way of eating as a few of the benefits of fasting. It is also important to note that intermittent fasting is not just a diet. It is a lifestyle change where you eat specifically during a set period of time, and you go without eating for another set period. Depending on the results you want, you can make the window of time when you eat bigger or the window of time when you do not eat bigger.

Fasting is as old as humankind itself. It has long been touted for its health benefits for the body and spiritual wellness. The benefits of fasting are hard-wired into our body as a biological mechanism against sickness. Think about the last time you were very sick. Did you want to eat? Of course not! As a matter of fact, when you ate, you probably wanted to throw up any of the food you ate. Hence, fasting is a biologic way to protect one's body when you are sick. Not only as an automatic biologic response to sickness, when you look into ancient history, but fasting was also a well-known remedy for illnesses. Greek philosophers often considered intermittent fasting as a solution to getting better. The Ancient era documents how many doctors prescribe fasting as a way to deal with illness. Despite the lack of modern tools, it is absolutely amazing how doctors knew that fasting and its different variations were a sure-fire way to deal with illnesses.

Additionally, fasting is a common solution to increase concentration or devoutness in the spiritual realm. Ezra Taft Benson, an American politician, and religious leader was right on the money when describing the mental and health benefits of intermittent fasting. Lots of religions practice some form of fasting as a way to connect with the Divine. Christians have fasted as a way to clean mental fogginess and realign their spiritual purpose. Muslims fast every year during Ramadan as a form of spiritual cleansing. Others have used fasting to make political statements which shows the power of fasting has on others as a show of solidarity for important issues that one believes in. Some cultures like Italians and other European countries usually have a heavy lunch and light breakfast or dinner, which as a form of intermittent fasting. Italians are often lauded worldwide for their diet with many others trying to emulate it in their day-to-day life. As you can see, fasting has been everywhere and is an important part of the human experience.

What intermittent fasting superior to other dieting methods is that it is a lifestyle. Unlike following a diet for a short of time to see limited results, intermittent fasting is a lifestyle choice that one follows every day. The main purpose of a diet is often times to lose weight. However, with intermittent fasting losing weight is only one benefit of the intermittent fasting lifestyle. Intermittent fasting has numerous benefits with weight loss only being an extra. Intermittent fasting has been linked to improving mental health, chronic illness, and heart disease, even helping to prevent certain cancers and seizures. Lifestyle change and extended health benefits are what makes intermittent fasting superior to other diets and methods.

The best thing about intermittent fasting is, once you get into the habit of doing it, the health results stay with you for years. You do not have to worry about getting into the horrible cycle of gaining weight and losing weight. Intermittent fasting is a habit that is inherently healthy and easier for one to maintain over long periods because it is something that you do every day without having to think about it. You can also mold it to fit the most hectic or most laid-back lifestyles.

While science is still studying all the benefits of intermittent fasting, the best thing about intermittent fasting is that ancient people already knew about the results. Whether to heal sickness or increase mental and spiritual well-being, intermittent fasting is a multi-tier approach to healing your entire body. Now is the time to touch base with the wisdom of our forefathers and get back to this lifestyle that has shown to be beneficial to our human ancestors and modern people alike. If you are looking for a way to improve your body and mind at the same time, then intermittent fasting is what you are looking for to do so. If done correctly, it is as safe as other diet methods and has the potential to stick with you a lot longer than fad dieting.

There are many reasons that people decide to fast. The main draw for many is the potential to lose weight. Fasting does not just help you lose weight, but it helps you to lose weight in one of the most stubborn places - your stomach. How many of us have struggled to try to lose those love handles and that muffin top! Never fear, intermittent fasting is the solution that you've been looking for to tackle these spots. Because intermittent fasting inherently restricts your meals to a certain time, you are already lowering your daily caloric intake. When you do that, you end up losing weight. However, intermittent fasting is more effective because it causes your weight loss hormones to rev up. When you are in a fasted state, your body gets energy from your body's fat stores and not the food that you are eating. This, in turn, increases your metabolism rate.

So, what is your metabolism rate? That is the rate at which you lose calories. You can lose calories by either eating less food or getting your body to use your stored fat, which is what intermittent fasting does. A definite win-win. Additionally, intermittent fasting helps you not to lose that much muscle compared to just fasting. When you still have some type of muscle on your body, your muscles work harder than fat to increase your metabolism, so you are losing weight while doing limited activities. When your muscles are used to this time of method of eating, you are essentially eating your way to losing weight, which is extremely helpful in the long-term of trying to maintain a healthy weight and healthy lifestyle. Another hormone that is affected by intermittent fasting is leptin. This hormone tells your brain which then tells your body when you are hungry. If you are obese, this hormone is overactive. Your body reads this hunger cue no matter if you are hungry or not which cause you to overeat. Thus, extra food and energy make you gain weight. When you fast, it helps improve your leptin sensitivity, so your body is more in tune with your hunger triggers, like ghrelin.

Intermittent fasting sends your brain more measured indicators of your hunger, so you are not overeating. However, it is important to stick to a pattern of fasting, especially if you are intermittent fasting, to avoid an increase of cortisol, which can lead to more stress or insomnia if you are not consistent with your fasting window.

Another reason people fast is to control type 2 diabetes. Diabetes is a chronic illness that occurs when a person's body is not able to send glucose, or blood sugar to your body. Glucose is what your body eat and to get that glucose your body needs insulin. People with type 1 diabetes do not produce insulin at all. Whereas people with type 2 diabetes produce insulin, but their bodies don't use insulin as efficiently as it should. As type 2 diabetes progresses, people tend not to make insulin at all.

Dr. Jason Fung did a study where 3 men fasted for a time frame of 10 months. Two of the men fasted every other day. And one man fasted three days a week. On the days that the men fasted, they were able to have low-calorie drinks like coffee, tea, and water. They could also have one low-calorie meal. At the end of the study, two of the men did not take any of their diabetes drugs. The last man had stopped taking four out of the five drugs that he was taking to control his diabetes. Dr. Fung asserts that fasting can be helpful for those with type 2 diabetes. However, other doctors caution against people taking this study as the complete truth since the study was only limited to three people. Nevertheless, the results seem quite promising. The most important thing from this study was Dr. Jason Fung demonstrated that fasting does have a positive effect on controlling diabetes. In the future, fasting will most likely be used as an important way to regulate, if not cure, type 2 diabetes.

An important consideration before fasting it to remember that if you are taking medication for your type 2 diabetes, you need to check in with your physician before attempting to fast to control your type 2 diabetes.

Another reason people choose to fast is to improve their physical appearance. Fasting reduces oxidative stress. To know more about oxidative stress, there must be a quick definition of what free radicals are. Free radicals are atoms in your body that are unstable. The free radicals have to join two other substances in your body to get stable. When free radicals join with other substances in your body, it causes oxidative stress. Hence, oxidative stress can cause cells to break down in your body and can result in issues such as inflammation and wrinkles and diseases or even chronic diseases. When you fast, it helps your body prevent forming these free radicals that can destroy your body in so many ways. Intermittent fasting also increases the human growth hormone which increases your body's collagen production. More collagen means that your body will have younger-looking skin. Moreover, fasting increases the process of autophagy, which is how your body repairs itself by making newer and healthier cells. When you have newer and healthier cells, your skin improves.

Fasting also helps the fluid that accumulates under the skin lessen, which also improves your overall appearance since salt is eliminated from your body when you fast. Less salt in your body increases your appearance and slows down the aging process.

The last major benefit of fasting that will be explored in this chapter is when people fast to improve their heart health. High blood pressure, cholesterol, diabetes, and obesity are all indicators of heart health problems. Fasting helps reduce all of these risks. However, fasting can cause an imbalance of your electrolytes, so when a person fasts, they must make sure that they are consuming enough electrolytes not to affect their heart health negatively. More about electrolytes will be discussed later in the book.

Before the chapter ends, a word of caution must be given. Some people should not fast. Those include people that have a history of eating disorders, pregnant women, breastfeeding women, teenagers, children and those with type 1 diabetes. Those with chronic illness or even cancers should also consult with their doctors before fasting.

The rule of thumb is to always consult with any health professional before you begin fasting. While it is great to have the desire to want to do intermittent fasting, before you begin, you will first want to check with your health professional before embarking on the fasting journey no matter if you are healthy or not. This is important to make sure you are fasting healthily and safely. Fasting should not make you feel sick. You will feel hunger, but if at any point, you begin to feel weird while fasting or run into any issues, keep an open line of communication open with your doctor or preferred health care provider.

Now that you know all the benefits and history of fasting, it's time to get to the meat and potatoes of the book – how to fast! Turn the page to learn more.

Chapter 2: How to Fast

Now that we have discusses the background of fasting, it's now important to offer practical advice about getting started. This chapter is dedicated to giving you tips that can help you deal with your hunger and survive the fasting process. Attention will be given to different fasts that are possible, including intermittent and other fasts. We will end with a list of fluids that you must have in order to deal with fasting long-term. There are three steps that you can take to get started.

Some people think that you need a lot of time and a big budget to get started intermittent fasting. The truth is that you don't need any of those things. You just need the determination and willpower to begin. Essentially, you can get started with three easy steps.

1. **Choose which fasting method you want to follow**. There are lots of different methods of fasting you can select from. Once you choose one, stick to it and begin the process. Do not feel obligated to continue a fasting method if you know that your body is responding negatively. You can always select a different method to follow.

2. **Calculate your calories and make sure you have a well-balanced diet.** Create a meal plan. Decide if you want to be vegetarian or vegan for more intense results. Do not underestimate the importance of counting your calories. Taking the time to plan your meals and make sure your calories are not going over your daily caloric count or under by too much will be the difference to being able to intermittent fasting correctly or not. Some people eat too much or too little. Do not be that person who fasts, but is still unhealthy.

3. **Decide which exercise you want to follow on the days that you are not fasting.** If you are going to exercise while fasting, make sure that you choose methods that are conducive to your fasting days. Take it easy on the days that you are fasting and go harder on the days that you are not fasting. If you need a little extra boost for the days you work out, try carbohydrate loading which is bulking up your meals with carbohydrates to help you make it through your workout. For longer fasts, do not worry about trying to exercise while fasting.

The rest of the book will go into more details about these three different steps. Feel free to take notes so you can come back and read your highlighted info. Don't feel pressure to be perfect from day one immediately. This lifestyle is a process, and you can slowly acclimate yourself to it. When you put unnecessary pressure on yourself, you add unneeded stress which can delay or hamper your results. Remember this is supposed to be fun and it's supposed to be about being a healthier person. Staying happy and positive will ensure that you will be fasting for years to come.

Choose Your Intermittent Fasting Method

Once you have figured out which fasting method you want to choose, the next thing you need to do before you begin intermittent fasting is to determine why you want to begin in the first place. What is your why? Why is it so important for you to start intermittent fasting? This can be a number of different reasons. Are you doing intermittent fasting in order to lose weight? Are you doing intermittent fasting to lead a healthier lifestyle? Are you doing intermittent fasting for another specific health outcome, like to lower your blood pressure or cholesterol levels or to even increase your metabolism or energy?

Whatever your reason is before beginning, make that reason clear so you can always come back to it as a point of reference when you feel like you are getting weak at any moment.

While your weight loss and health journey are different than other people's, it is interesting to look at other people who fast to see what they're doing and what works for them. You can use them as inspiration. You can also form your own support group to hold you accountable for your reasons for intermittent fasting. You can find this support group online or in person, like a family member or trusted friend. Checking out online boards every now and then is also great to do in order to keep your info up-to-date and to recharger your intermittent fasting battery. If you are unable to find such a support group around, don't be afraid to start your own.

Imagine how fun it will be to have a group of people supporting each other and knowing that you started it. People tend to be social and love to work out in groups. And intermittent fasting group can be a unique way to encourage yourself and encourage others and help a group of people get healthy at the same time. Popular places to look for people interested in such a group would be Craigslist, meetup.com, or even putting flyers in local coffee shops, doctor's offices or the library. Don't be shy if there isn't a group. It may be a sign that you are the one that is needed to start such a group.

The next thing you want to do before you begin is to speak with your doctor. When you meet, let your doctor know what your reasons for wanting to do intermittent fasting are. Then see if they have any input. This especially important if you have diabetes, are elderly or pregnant or have a history of eating disorders. If you fall into any of these categories, do not skip this step. The doctor can give you certain steps to avoid as well as give you some tips on how to take your results to the next level. Keeping your doctor aware of what you're doing can make sure that you always have a health professional in your corner and support to give insights when you need it.

The next important step you should do before you begin is to have realistic expectations. If you plan on losing 50 pounds in a week, that's most likely not going to happen. It is healthy to lose at least two pounds a week. Even if you have a realistic expectation of how much weight you want to lose, what happens if you are not seeing the results you think you should be seeing? (We'll talk about this some in the next chapter.) The most important point about your expectations is to adjust them. You may not meet your expectations, and that is ok. You can adjust your expectations or adjust your actions to meet them. Do not get discouraged if you do not meet your expectations. Keep going! You do not want to throw in the towel too soon or throw the towel in without adjusting your expectations. No matter what your expectations are, continue to arm yourself with the proper information by researching so, you can see how intermittent fasting best fits into your lifestyle. When you have your reasons for doing intermittent fasting and your food journal ready, you can go ahead and begin.

Schedule your Day of Reckoning. This is the day where you get rid of everything in your kitchen that's not going to help you with your intermittent fasting journey. These items are things like junk food, alcohol, snacks, salty and sugary drinks. Sugary drinks include diet drinks and health drinks like Gatorade or Powerade. These all contain fructose which is just as deadly and inflammation causing as sugar. You can give those bad foods to a friend or family member, a food bank or just throw them away. For the more dramatic people like me, you can even burn them. This day of reckoning is a special day in your intermittent fasting journey. It is the day of no return, and it can symbolically signify your new lifestyle is an intermittent faster. This step can be as fun or as dramatic as you would like it. However, once you choose this day stick with it, so you know it's time to begin a new way of life.

Next thing is, like Nike, 'Just do it!' Pick your fasting window and eating time and start. Initially, do not expect just to go 24 hours without food, definitely build up to that goal. When you start off slow, you can try to avoid maybe eating breakfast since you already sleeping and coming from a fast. Another way to get a slow start is if you try to reduce the portions of a certain food that you are eating before you totally give up the food that you are eating. For example, if you just have to have 10 cokes a day. Trying have 5, then 3, then 1, until you are at zero.

Other ways to go incrementally fast are to change perhaps the portion of the food that you are eating. If you are used to eating carbohydrate-heavy meals, slowly change your diet to include more fruits and vegetables until your portions start to consist of mostly vegetables and whole foods. If you eat more white bread or grain products, work on not eating them or even substituting them for healthier options like sprouted slices of bread or wheat or brown carbohydrates. This incremental beginning can help you be more successful when you ramp up to more intense versions of intermittent fasting such as skipping days at a time.

Once you begin fasting, you can start journaling and keeping track of what you are eating. I like to use an old-fashioned pen and paper to track my daily meals in a food journal. However, one of the easiest ways to keep track of your calories and food choices is by using technology. Since our phones are already near us, you can easily use your phone as a resource to help you with your intermittent fasting journey. You can use your phone to choose an app that helps with your fasting. A couple of the most popular choices include Body Fasting app or Fitness Pal. Some apps have extra bonuses you can use, like hiring a personal health coach for extra support.

As you keep track of your journey, do not forget to take note of your victories! Celebrate them. Perhaps you've been fasting three days in a row and are on track to fat perfectly for a week! Celebrate that! When you are tracking your food, take notes of certain trends. Are you meeting your calorie guidelines? Do you notice any trends about when you are mindlessly snacking or eating because you are stressed or because you didn't plan your meals well? Being able to track this information can help you create practices to help you combat your weaknesses.

On the other hand, if you end up going over on your calorie count one day, that's ok. The next day is a new day, and you should just get back on track and do not get too bogged down if you do not meet your goal. Your journal will also help you see if you are being serious or not. You may trick other people, but you cannot fool yourself. Your journal will reflect if you need to give yourself a stern talking to or if you are being committed to being healthy or not. While what you eat is very important to maintaining your intermittent fasting lifestyle, it is not the only important thing. You should also make sure that you are getting enough sleep and exercising as well. If you like to bedazzle your personal items, now is the time to do it. Personalize your journal so that it's your own. Because it's going to be an important part of your intermittent fasting journey.

The longer you stay up, the more chances you have of eating more food. Sleeping helps with your fasting, and it also helps keep your cortisol levels low. Cortisol is a hormone that helps regulate your sleep. High levels of cortisol can potentially lead to insomnia. Intermittent fasting helps you sleep more peacefully, calmly and through the night. And by sleeping, it helps with your fasting a mutually beneficial relationship. When you add in exercise to the intermittent fasting equation, it only helps you have a better night's rest as well as compounding your intermittent fasting results.

Calculate Your Calories

One of the major tricks of being successful at fasting is to make sure that you have meals prepared so you will not be tempted to eat things that aren't good for you or overeat. In order to get those meals prepared ahead of time, you will want to have a pantry of your necessities in order to get those meals planned, but you have no idea how to begin.

The first thing we will discuss is the approach to take. The first approach is easy. Since you already eat certain foods on a daily basis, find healthier recipes for the meals that you are already eating. The next way is to build your meals ahead of time. When planning a meal, you can try to have three different colors – a fruit, veggie, bean or a whole-wheat grain. You will also want to try to cook foods a healthy way like steaming, baking or roasting instead of frying and grilling. Cooking at home will definitely help you save more calories than eating out. (However, if you must eat out, look for the healthiest alternatives you can find.)

One way to prepare your meals ahead of time is to assemble the ingredients and freeze them. So when it is time to make your meal, you can thaw the ingredients and make them. Another way to prepare your meals ahead of time is to prepare your entire meal, like casseroles or easily freezable recipes, and then un-thaw them ahead of time and prepare them. As you start to fast more and more, you will discover what meals are your favorites and which meals are the easiest to prepare.

To give you an idea of what types of healthy ingredients you can stock up on before you being meal planning follows.

- **Proteins** - Beans, quinoa, lean meats, nuts, peanut butter or your favorite type of nut butter

- **Vegetables** – Kale, spinach, lettuce, broccoli, mixed veggies, (The more vegetables you have, the merrier!)

- **Fiber** – Oatmeal, lettuce

- **Fruit** – Fresh, canned and frozen. Be careful of the sugar content in canned and frozen fruits to make sure unnecessary sugar is not being added.

- **Healthy fats** – Nuts, seeds, olive oil and coconut oil, oily fish like salmon and tuna

- **Carbohydrates** – brown rice, wheat loaves of bread and sprouted slices of bread

- **Vitamins** – Fish oil, Vitamin C, your favorite brand of all-purpose vitamins

You want to eat whole foods that contain lots of macronutrients. Macronutrients you want in your food include carbohydrates, fat, protein, minerals, vitamins, and water. I also want to make fiber an honorable mention. When you eat food with high levels of fiber, your digestive health improves. A simple rule of thumb is to keep your plate with as many varied colors as possible. Foods to consider eating are going to be lots of leafy vegetables like kale, swiss chard, greens, and lettuce; dark fruit like blackberries, raspberries, and strawberries, and drink lots of water even if you are already drinking lots of water. You can look into getting protein from non-meat sources such as nuts, quinoa or beans.

Do not forget to avoid worthless calories or foods that do not contain many nutrients that will keep you full, especially foods with lots of sugar. Sugar is everywhere! It is one of the most difficult things to cut out of your diet. However, if you want intermittent fasting to work, you will definitely want to be diligent against sugar. An ingredient to look for would be ingredients that end in "-ose," or anything that says, "high fructose corn syrup." Easy ways to give up sugar is to gradually get rid of them by eliminating the most obvious culprits that have a high sugar count such as candy, soda (diet or otherwise), or juice.

Also, giving up carbohydrates helps you rid yourself of the sugar. By eating whole foods with a dense nutrient count, it will help you avoid those cravings until you no longer even want sugar. While alcohol is not forbidden, it is one of those foods that take up calories without giving you many nutrients in return. Also, be mindful of those sneaky sugar calories in workout drinks or salty post-workout snacks that do not really help you enjoy the benefits of your workout! Additionally, when you go out to eat, try to have a peek at the menu in advance and try to pick out the options that fit into your calorie count.

Other quick notes to remember are:

- **Snacks and drinks add extra calories to your meal** so be mindful of what you are eating and drinking throughout the day. Are you eating and drinking because you are hungry or because you are bored?

- **Make a grocery list and prep for the week.** This will save you time and money!

- **Have fun searching for recipes.** To add some variety to your menu, try new ones! Being healthy is a positive so have fun with it! Your meal planning is adjustable, so you do not have to feel boxed in.

- **When you meal prep, do not feel like you have to do everything in one day.** You can cut your vegetables one day, and make your sauces on the next day. You can also go ahead and prepare the ingredients, even the spices you are going to use beforehand, so the cooking will be seamless.

One way to amplify the benefits of fasting is if you pair your fasting with a vegan or vegetarian diet. Vegan diets consume no animal products such as eggs or honey. Vegetarians do not consume any meat, but they are allowed to eat eggs and products made by animals. Another popular diet to pair your intermittent fasting with is the ketogenic diet.

The ketogenic diet is rich in proteins, fats and limits carbohydrates. This diet is great and trying to prevent seizures as well. Even if you do not want to partake in one of these diets, the intermittent lifestyle is still great for you. As long as you are staying within your caloric limit for the day and within your fasting window, you are ok. You can incorporate it into your lifestyle not matter if you cook at home or go out to eat.

If you want to go vegetarian or vegan, here a few tips that can help!

- For dairy milk, you can substitute any type of non-dairy milk like almond milk, soy milk or cashew milk. You can also make your own milk by soaking cashews in water overnight and then blending the cashews with water and adding extracts like vanilla or almond or whichever you prefer to give it extra flavor.

- For recipes that require yogurt, you can look into substituting a vegan alternative for yogurt.

- Butter, mayonnaise, cheese or cream cheese can be substituted for any vegan brand of the same product.

- There are many different ways to substitute eggs. You can use tofu instead of eggs if you are looking for a scrambled texture. If you are using eggs to bind items in a recipe, you can use unsweetened applesauce, soft tofu, mashed bananas or the popular flax seed egg, which is just 1 tablespoon of ground flax seeds plus 3 tablespoons of water or another liquid and blend it all together. Then add the flax egg to the recipe.

- For meaty textures, you can try tofu. Use seitan or meatless meat. You can also use mushrooms or cauliflower, instead of meat, or even blended nuts to give it the same meaty texture.

- Instead of using honey, you can use agave, maple syrup, or any type of plant-based sweetener.

- There are also many different types of fish substitutions. You can search for your favorite vegan fish substitute to still enjoy fish recipes. Thankfully, there are a lot of vegan substitutes that are divine. When you incorporate them into your recipes, you won't be able to notice that you are having a vegetarian or vegan dish because it is as good as a dish with meat.

What Exercise Will You Incorporate?

To determine what's the best exercise regimen for you to incorporate into your lifestyle, remember your why. Again, your goals will help you determine which exercise regime is best. No matter what exercise you do, it is recommended that you get at least 30 minutes of active exercise every day or 150 minutes a week to keep your heart healthy.

If you do not have money for a gym membership or personal trainer, one of the easiest ways to get a workout in, is to look for exercise routines online, especially on YouTube. There are a lot of free workouts on there. If you are sedentary most of the time and have a little extra money to spend, you can invest in a desk peddler or a standing desk so you can move while you are working. Another quick way to work out is just to do those basic old-fashioned exercises that you used to do in grade school, such as push-ups, sit-ups, jumping rope, and jumping jacks for thirty minutes. However, the key to this type of workout is to go as fast as you can and perform the exercises in sets. Perhaps you can do 3 sets of one exercise, rest, then do another three set of exercises and rest and keep going until you reach your 30 minutes.

Exercise is something you definitely want to incorporate into your intermittent lifestyle if you want to maintain results and if you want to live in overall health or life. Do not make excuses. Find a way to be active!

Of course, when you first start off fasting, you may take some time to get adjusted. To assist in meeting your weight loss goals, you may want to use a calorie counter. An easy way to track your calories throughout the day is to use a food journal. In the food journal, you will want to you notate the calories that you are consuming and the nutrient breakdown to make sure that you are meeting your goals. The more specific or strict you are can determine how quickly you meet your health close. A food journal will also help you notice trends. What do you do before you eat bad foods usually? What are your cravings? Do they only happen on certain days or when you eat certain foods? Are you drinking enough water every day? These are all tips that can help you eat healthily and a great tool to pair with your fasting. This will be a valuable tool as you begin to get into the habit of intermittent fasting.

If you need a little extra support, do not be afraid to look into health apps that offer health coaching. That may just be the extra boost you need. Health apps are truly popular and growing every day. You will be sure to find one that you need as long as you do a quick search on the App Store.

Do not be alarmed if you ever run into bumps. The key is to pick right back up where you left off. This chapter is a great one to come and visit for reference. We started off with three steps to help you get started intermittent fasting. You went over planning your meals, stocking your pantry, and making sure you are reaching your daily caloric limit, so you do not under eat or ovary.

The chapter also goes deeper into exercises you can incorporate to take your intermittent fasting to the next level. More importantly, this chapter offers some insight about what to do if you run into any plateaus or any issues while you are intermittent fasting. They are bound to happen, but the key is to keep going. Do not get discouraged. We all make mistakes. Have a short memory and pick up the next day if you are ever to fall short. A major tool for making your fasting journey work is the food journal that you should be keeping. Whether it is a hard copy or digital copy, a meal journal is key so you can know your personal trends and figure out the best practices that will work for you as you fast.

Now, what about all those fasting methods we keep talking about? We'll begin talking about intermittent fasting first.

Intermittent fasting is eating during certain windows and then not eating during other windows. It may sound complicated, but it's really not. Most people have done some sort of fasting without even knowing. The easiest way to practice intermittent fasting is to skip the meal that is easiest for you according to your current schedule. This version is called spontaneous fasting. Maybe you are in a rush and forget to eat breakfast. You just intermittently fasted! Perhaps you are preparing for a busy meeting and decide to skip lunch. Yup, you just intermittently fasted.

Spontaneous intermittent fasting is very easy to do, and many often partake in it without knowing it. To make this method more effective, instead of missing a meal by accident, you will miss it purposefully. If you are already doing this accidentally, then you can just fine tune it so it can become your official intermittent fasting method. This is definitely one of the easiest methods to do since it happens without you thinking about it. However, there are other methods that you can definitely consider, as well.

The next version of intermittent fasting is called The Warrior Diet. When you practice this version of intermittent fasting, you only eat small pieces of raw fruits and vegetables during the day and eat one major meal at night. The major meal you eat should be limited to about 500-600 calories for women and 800-900 calories for men. Muslims practice a form of this intermittent fasting version during Ramadan when they forgo eating during the day and only eat after sunset.

Every other day fasting is when you fast every other day. During this version of fasting, you eat a limited amount of meals during your off days and on the days that you are allowed to eat you just eat regularly. A similar version of this intermittent fasting method is called the 5:2. During this method, you eat for 5 full days, and you fast for 2 days by only eating a total of 500 to 600 calories on the days that you are fasting. For women, if you are using this method, it is advised that you eat 500 calories, and for men, it is advised that you eat 600 calories. You can break your smaller meals into two meals of 300 calories or 250 calories respectively. The trick when using this method is to eat the same amount as you would if you were eating regularly on the days that you can eat.

You also do not want to fast for two days in a row, especially for women. It is advised that you break up the fasting days during the week so that the two fasting days are not one after the other. With this intermittent fasting method, it is extremely important to meal plan to make sure that you are reaching your caloric limit. This method requires that you are vigilant about your meal planning so that you are not overeating or undereating. This method can definitely be more challenging to start with, but once you get into the habit of doing it, it will become a lot easier.

One of the most popular versions of intermittent fasting is called the 16/8 fast. While you do this type of fast, you only eat during an 8 to 10-hour window and then you fast the other 16 hours of the day. Popular times to fast can be from 10 am to 6 pm, or 9 am to 5 pm, or even 11 am to 7 pm. This method of fasting is beneficial because you are able to follow your natural hunger cycles. Some people are never hungry in the morning, so they are able to forgo breakfast. Some people do not like to eat after a certain amount of time in the evening, so they forego dinner. By using this method of fasting, you are able to add intermittent fasting to your lifestyle without having to make a major adjustment. To take this method to the next level, some people fast for 20 hours and only eat during a 4-hour window.

The more you fast, the more you can potentially lose weight as long as you are making sure that you are eating healthy during your eating times. One of the most difficult intermittent fasting methods is called the 24-hour fast. Some people fast from dinner one day to the end of the next day or breakfast one day to breakfast the next day. For beginners, it is probably best to start off with a smaller window and work your way up to not eating for longer periods of time. Only the most advanced, most determined fasters should try this initially. This method also requires lots of willpower and self-control. People, who are new to intermittent fasting, read this and think, "Who in the world is trying this method of intermittent fasting?" Sure, actors and actresses may use this method to get ready for movie roles, but a lot of regular people use it, too. You will be surprised that it is very convenient for lots of people to follow. As you become more versed with intermittent fasting, you may find that you too that prefer The Warrior Diet over different methods of intermittent fasting.

Another popular intermittent fasting, one that has the most research done on it, is the every-other-day fast, or the Alternate Daily Fasting (ADF). Don't let the name fool you. Alternate daily fasting is similar to the 5:2 diet in that you can eat up to 500 calories on the days that you fast. The only difference is that you fast on alternate days rather than 2 times a week like in the 5:2 diets. Intermittent fasting is usually less than 24 hours, but there are those who have had smashing success with longer diets, specifically, 24 hours, 36 hours, 42 hours and 2 weeks fasts. We will examine these in more detail later in the book. You will be surprised that the longer one fasts, the less hungry they get. You will also realize that longer fasts are not impossible, and if you can successfully get through one, you may realize how awesome it is. We will talk about longer fasts in the next chapter.

So what about hunger? You will get hungry at some point while fasting, but you will be able to overcome. Intermittent fasting takes advantage of our body's natural cycle of breaking down energy in our bodies. The way fasting works in the body is simple. Our bodies need the energy to run. When we eat, we receive energy from the foods we eat like beans, vegetables, fruits, and carbohydrates to name a few. Our bodies then take sugar or glucose from the food and keep it stored in the muscles and liver. When our bodies need energy, they release it into our bloodstream so our bodies can use it. Yet, when a person begins to fast, our bodies need to get the energy from a different source. After about eight hours of fasting, our livers use most of the glucose that is in our bodies. Our body then goes into gluconeogenesis, which indicates our body is about to enter fasting mode. When a person's body is in gluconeogenesis, this means that the calories that their body burns increases because if the body doesn't have any energy coming it, it makes its own glucose using your body fat. Once the body runs out of fat to use, it then begins to enter into starvation mode.

Starving people are in a severe bodily mode in which their body is essentially eating itself to provide nutrients. This mode takes an extended amount of days and months to reach. It is not something that you can enter easily after a few hours of not eating. Intermittent fasting takes advantage of the gluconeogenesis mode that allows your body to burn more calories. This sweet spot of gluconeogenesis is where the leverage of intermittent fasting lies. You can safely fast for three days with water only by yourself. If you want to fast longer than three days with water fast, be sure to touch base with your healthcare professional.

One of the major keys to surviving any fasting period is the importance of staying hydrated. It also helps you not enter starvation mode. Of course, you will want to drink water, but there are other liquids, you should be aware of. The key to drinking while fasting is to partake in drinks that have no calories. Here's a list of drinks you should consider drinking while fasting.

- **Water** - Water is one of the best liquids to consume while fasting. You can add a slice of lemon or infuse it with herbs, like basil, mint, or your favorite fruit. It is important to stay away from any sweeteners that can mess up your fast. This means you want to avoid sugary water enhancers like Crystal Light or any type of artificial flavoring to give the water more flavor. Enjoy the water as I,s and let it help you make it through the fast. To make your water fancier, you may even want to consider sparkling water. Mineral water is also great to drink during your fast.

- **Broth -** Any type of vegetable or bone -flavored broth can help you make it through a fast. If you can, you want to stay away from the store-bought broth that will have lots of extra sodium and flavors the best thing to do is to make your own broth. The broth is really helpful when you are fasting for longer than 24 hours.

- **Tea -** Any type of tea has proved to be extremely beneficial when you are fasting. Oolong, herbal, black, and green tea are all great to drink while you are fasting. Generally, tea improves your gut digestion, cellular detox, and balance of your probiotics. Be sure to watch the caffeine intake with the teas. It's good to go for caffeine-free options like ginger, chamomile, lemongrass, and hibiscus. You don't want to get addicted to caffeine or use it too much tea as an appetite suppressant while you are fasting. Peppermint tea helps get rid of your bloating and gas. Cinnamon chai tea is great to bust any sugar cravings you may have. Oolong and black tea lower your blood sugar. Lastly, green tea is great for an appetite suppressant.

- **Apple cider vinegar** - This is another type of liquid that can be very helpful during your fasting period as it helps improve your digestion and can help suppress your appetite.

- **Coffee** - Another great liquid to have during your fast is coffee. If you drink coffee, you want to make sure it does not cause an upset stomach or cause a racing heart. If drinking coffee does this to you, you may consider not drinking it. When drinking coffee in your fast, you also want to avoid using any artificial sweeteners, milk, or cream that will add extra calories. Avoid butter and coconut oil, too.

  If you want to flavor your coffee, consider adding spices like cinnamon, nutmeg or ginger for the bowl people.

- **Smoothies** - Smoothies are another great way to get the nutrition that you need. You can add vegetables to get the most out of your diet.

- **Pureed Soups** - These are great as well. You can even consider pureeing your favorite low-calorie meal if you want to stick to the liquid fast. This is another way you can get the nutrients that you need.

Now for the bad. Drinks that you should want to stay away from are sugary sodas, coconut water, juices, workout drinks like Gatorade or Powerade and definitely energy drinks. Almond milk is also a beverage you want to avoid while fasting. All these drinks have extra calories which will null-and-void your fast.

One more important thing to know about liquids is that it can help you beat symptoms of hunger while you are fasting. If you are having issues with dizziness or headaches, you will want to drink more water. Mineral water is also great for both of these issues. If you are having muscle cramps, you will want to drink water and soak in an Epsom salt bath to soak in. You may also consider taking a magnesium supplement.

Lastly, if you are experiencing constipation, eat more fiber and drink more water during your eating period. You'll want to have more fruits, vegetables, and even chia seeds that have been soaked in a liquid like almond milk or even water if you're watching your calories. As long are you are consuming food during your eating windows, you will be ok. The next chapter will go into more detail about things to look out for when fasting and how to take the leap into extending fasting times.

Chapter 3: Frequently Asked Questions And some Fasting Tips

When you begin fasting, it is important to make notes in your food journal. It will give insights on how you can manage your fasts better and longer. So when you get super-duper hungry, and you do not know how to stop your hunger, you'll look at your food journal. Your food journal notes will help you see what cravings you are normally having? Are you eating whole foods and foods with lots of fiber? Do you notice any other trends or have tried any other recipes to help with your hunger? If so, some other ways to curb your hunger pangs are:

- Distract yourself! Sometimes you have to focus on something else so you will not focus on the hunger.

- Learning how to deal with your hunger pangs. Initially, you are going to feel hungry. If you can train your mind that it will last only a little while, and they typically do, you will be able to pick right back up and make it to your next meal.

- Consider avoiding snacks. There have been people to say that snacking throughout the day helps to lose weight. The truth is that the total number of calories determine whether if you lose weight. So if you are a snacker and you need them to function, continue to do so as long as the snack does not interfere with your daily calorie count. However, try to take them out and just eat the main meals during your eating period to see if you notice a difference or not.

- When you eat, make sure you are chewing at least 30 times before you swallow. This makes sure that you are properly digesting your food, enjoying the flavors, and slowing down your meal to make sure you are not overeating.

- Also stopped eating a little bit before you feel complete and drink water. This is another good tip to help you prevent overeating.

- Next, try not to sleep after you eat. This won't help you as you try to become more efficient with fasting. It will actually hinder your progress.

- Drink lots of water and do not forget to take your vitamins. Water is an important way to intermittent fast successfully.

Fasting is indeed a lifestyle, and there are a few mistakes you want to be aware of once you begin. Knowing what they are beforehand will hopefully help you not to have to struggle with them at all. Even if you run into any bumps in the road, remember to get right back up and to keep going. You are not expected to be perfect the first time you try your hand at. With careful planning and perseverance, you will be intermittent fasting like a pro in no time. These are some of the top mistakes that people make while they are intermittent fasting. Take notes and try to avoid them if you can.

- **Over-eating and binge-eating** – Avoiding overeating and binge eating during eating time are crucial in intermittent fasting. When it is time to eat, eat a regular sized portion and do not try to compensate for your fasting period. This overcompensation prevents you from taking advantage of your intermittent fasting period.

- **Not eating enough** - When you eat, do not feel like you can't eat. Take advantage of your eating period, but do not gorge yourself. Make sure you are eating healthy food and not junk. If you make sure your food is full of macronutrients, you will be able to make it through your fasted states easier.

- **Not drinking enough water** – Water is the life force of us all and staying hydrated is a major key to making the intermittent lifestyle work for you. Staying hydrated prevents cravings and helps you make it through the fasting period. Do not neglect this important step.

- **Not choosing the right method** – Intermittent fasting should be easy. If it feels like you have to work too much or it is not flowing with your lifestyle, do not be afraid to try a new method. There is not a hard and fast rule about which method is the best. Whichever method you choose should fit into your lifestyle. Remember, this is a lifestyle change and not a diet. You can take the time to figure out which method works the best for you.

- **Obsessing too much** - If you are weighing yourself obsessively or worrying about if you are doing intermittent fasting, take a deep breath and relax. Results can take time. You shouldn't expect a drastic change overnight. Just relax and take your time. Before you know it, you will see the benefits that are extremely helpful.

- **Giving up too soon** – Do not join the many other people who threw in the towel too soon on intermittent fasting. Give yourself about two weeks to measure the results and see if it is working or not. Do not just give up after a day or two. This method is proven throughout time to work. This tricky part is finding which method works out the best for you. Keep playing around with it and do not give up too soon. However, if, at any point, you being to experience drastic results, it may be time to throw in the towel.

Ultimately, if you are food journaling, you will be able to pick up on some of these mistakes that you make. Any time you noticed a mistake, try to find a way to correct it with better practice. Be gentle and kind to yourself and keep going. You will soon realize that intermittent fasting and fasting is not that bad.

Plateauing

After you start fasting, you may run into a few issues. You have lost a couple of pounds, but now you are not sure how to lose more. You've seemed to flatline. What do you do next? This section is all about how to maintain the weight you have lost and how to overcome any ruts you may run into.

First things first, here are a few questions to ask yourself about how to maintain your weight. When you initially start intermittent fasting, you may see huge results, but if at any time you begin to eat more and not exercise portion control, there is the chance you may gain that weight back. However, there are some ways to try and monitor your weight so you can stay on the straight-and-narrow intermittent path.

- When you look in your food journal or your calorie are you still eating the same amount of calories? Has that number changed at all? If so, why? And how can you fix it? What other weird trends do you notice? For example, on days that you are busy, you notice that you always break your fast? How can you fix some of the challenges on the trends that you see?

- Are you drinking enough water? Sometimes you are not hungry, you are dehydrated and drinking more water can prevent you from eating worthless calories.

- Are you binging during your meals when you can eat or are you eating normal potions? It is expected that you may gain some weight back if you are eating double portions to compensate for when you are not eating. The idea is to keep the same amount of food that you are eating so your body can reap the benefits of a true fasting period.

- Additionally, what types of foods are you eating? Has the method you have chosen fit easily into your current lifestyle or are you having a difficult time fasting with the current method you've chosen? Are you only eating carbohydrates like bread and pasta with limited fruits and vegetables? If you must have some of your favorite unhealthy foods, see if you can find a vegetarian or vegan or a healthier version of that recipe.

- Have you tried a different fasting window? A different fasting window sometimes can provide better results. You can play around with different fasting windows until you find the one that works the best for you.

- How is your sugar intake? Are you still eating sugar in high amounts or even eating foods that have those sneaky sugar calories hidden inside them? A review of the ingredients in the foods that you eat can help you find the culprit.

- Are there any days where you are feeling dizzy, nauseated, fatigued or having difficulty concentrating? What are the foods that you are eating when you notice these symptoms? This will help you figure out if the food you are eating is agreeable or if you need to eat more or less of certain foods.

- Are your meals well-balanced? Are you seeing a lot of different colors from different food groups on your plate when you eat or only one type of color?

- How fast did you transition to intermittent fasting? Are you getting enough calories for your energy needs? If you are drastically below the recommended count for women or men, you may need to eat more.

- Are you eating enough when you work out? Are you carb cycling which means you eat a slightly bigger portion on the days you work out to help you have a great workout versus the days when you do not work out.

- Are you having trouble binging on sugar or having a difficult time breaking bad habits? If so, perhaps you can allow yourself at least 3 cheat meals a month to satisfy those cravings.

- What type of exercises are you doing? Are the exercises complementary to weight or muscle gain? If the exercises you are doing are helping you gain muscle, like lifting weights, you may not be losing weight, but you are gaining muscle which can help you lose weight in the long term. More cardio based exercises can help you burn more calories and potentially lose more weight. Be sure to make sure your exercise regimen is helping you reach your goals.

Mind you, if you were to stop at all, you might gain some of the weight that you've lost. So keep going! Do not give up. The race is not to the swift but to those who endure, be mindful that you may not see changes because you are with your body all the time. However, if you ask someone else, they may be able to point out changes that you are not aware of so do not be afraid to ask for a second opinion.

Additionally, weight loss may not be the first benefits you see. Note your mood and your focus and your energy levels to see if intermittent fasting has made an impact on your life in other ways besides wait. Trust me, people will know and talk about it if they notice a difference. If they don't, that's okay too. Just ask for their honest opinion and see what they have to say if you need some validation. Just make sure the person that you're asking if someone that you trust and who has your best interest in mind.

Remember, if you do not see your expectations being met as quickly as you expect, it is okay to make a few changes to see if you can reach your goals. After tweaking a few things while you fast, and you still aren't meeting your expectations it may be time to get more realistic ones. Nevertheless, keep working with your intermittent fasting windows, your meal, and portion choices as well as your exercise routines until you get the results that you want. Mistakes and mishaps are inevitable, but it is important to keep a good sense of humor and a sense of determination so you can make it through.

Hopefully, this chapter has put to rest any fear that you may have about intermittent fasting and assured you of the benefits that it has. Even if you do not decide to stick with intermittent fasting long-term, at least giving it a try will open your eyes to a new method of living and your body will thank you. Hopefully, you are convinced about all the benefits of intermittent fasting and fasting! The last chapter will give you a few recipes you can use to start your intermittent and fasting journey.

Frequently Asked Questions

At this point, I am sure that you have a lot of questions that you need to be answered about fasting and myths that need to be busted. For those who are on the fence or those who are excited to begin, this section will be especially helpful. It will go over some common myths that may give you pause before beginning as well as alleviate some of the fears you may have. Hopefully, by the time you finish reading, you will be ready to get started fasting!

How do I get over the mental block of not eating?

If you do not eat, you feel like you are starving. Ever had this feeling? No worries, you are not alone. This is a common feeling to have. Sometimes when we get that feeling, it doesn't mean that we're always hungry. It can mean that you are thirsty instead. If you are having trouble overcoming this barrier, think about what you can do when you do get this feeling. What's your plan of action going to be? How about drinking a glass of water, listening to your favorite song or doing your favorite activity until the feeling passes? I'll be honest. The mental block of not being able to eat is one of the most difficult barriers overcome when doing intermittent fasting, but it is not difficult to overcome once you get in the habit of doing it. Once you make it through, you will realize that it will get easier and easier until your body gets used to the fasting period and your eating period.

There are a lot of questions that people have about intermittent fasting and the validity of how it can help improve your overall health. This chapter addresses some of the most common misconceptions and frequently asked questions one may have about intermittent fasting. Hopefully, after reading this chapter, if you are on the fence, you will be convinced about the positives about intermittent fasting.

What's the best diet to couple intermittent fasting with?

Great question. There is not an 'official' one. It depends on your goals. If you want to lose more weight, popular diets to pair with intermittent fasting are vegan, vegetarian or keto diets. More important than diet is the importance of eating a well-balanced diet not matter which dietary option you decide upon and stay within our caloric limits.

Can I use the ketogenic diet to intermittent fast if I am diabetic?

Some people have coupled intermittent fasting with a keto diet with some success. However, there are still studies being done to determine if this is the best way to do intermittent fasting with diabetes. There are some benefits to intermittent fasting with diabetes like regulation of your insulin and glycogen levels. However, the most important step is to talk with your healthcare provider before deciding to take this journey.

Is it safe?

Yes. For healthy adults, intermittent fasting should not be an issue. You may even realize that there are many more benefits to intermittent fasting than you thought. However, for those who are elderly, pregnant, breastfeeding or taking medication, check with your healthcare provider first.

How much can I train on an empty stomach?

The most difficult part of training while intermittent fasting is to let your body get used to it. When your body gets used to working out while fasting, you will realize that you may get extra strength and energy to do your workout. When you train while you fast, your workout can be more efficient and help you burn more calories or build more muscle. So if you can handle training on an empty stomach go for it. Ultimately, it is up to you and your exercise goals to decide what you can handle.

Many people decide to train during their eating window so they can eat a pre and post workout meal. If you are trying to lose weight, foregoing your pre-workout meal will greatly help. Just remember that after your work out, try to eat protein and fiber to rebuild your body from the workout. Others also find that eating more carbohydrates on the days that they work out, helps them with the workouts.

Can I just eat fruits as a main meal?

It is best to eat a balanced diet. Too much fruit could give you too much sugar and give you unwanted weight gain if you do it too often. If you prefer fruits, try to disguise your greens by adding your greens with your fruits in a juice blend or smoothie.

What are the side effects?

You may experience headaches, diarrhea, cramps, and discomfort. You may also experience insomnia, lower back pain, and hair loss. But if you experience these, reach out to your health care providers since these are extreme side effects. The most common side effects are hunger pangs, headaches, and discomfort. You should not feel totally lethargic or as if you cannot function by missing a meal or two a day. If you try intermittent fasting and you have just horrible side effects, it may not be for you, and that is okay.

How do I help with my hunger pangs?

One way to help with your hunger is to drink lots of liquid especially water. You can drink a big glass of water when you wake up or anytime you experience hunger pangs. What's more, you can put Himalayan salt in your water to give it an extra boost. You can also drink tea, amino acids, and coffee as much as you'd like, too. Just watch the extras like milk, cream, and sugar.

How can I tell if intermittent fasting or fasting is working?

One way to tell if it is working or not is to look at your body. Are you losing weight? How do you feel? Do you feel like you are sleeping better? Do you have a clearer mind or energy boost? Do you feel happiness generally? These are factors to look at when deciding if it is the right lifestyle for you or not. It is also important to note which method of intermittent fasting works best for you.

Why should I skip breakfast? Is not breakfast the most important meal of the day?
Wonderful question. The word breakfast means to break the fast. This idea that breakfast is the most important meal of the day is from an outdated diet concept. The typical American diet consists of sweet breakfast options like waffles, pancakes, pastries, etc. If you are not going to eat a healthy breakfast, why eat it anyway? Making sure you have enough calories throughout the day is more important than when you eat it. So if you eat your first meal at lunch, then your "breakfast" would be your "lunch."

Eating breakfast or not is totally up to your body and whether you and your body can handle it or not. The great thing is if you need breakfast to function, just make it a part of your eating window and make sure you are eating a healthy option for breakfast. Most people tend to skip breakfast, so that's why skipping breakfast is not a major issue for most people. However, listen to your body and do what's best for your body's natural cycle.

Is not it healthier to eat more meals throughout the day?

This is a great question, too. The nutrients in your food and the number of calories you are eating is more important than when you eat it. If your body responds to smaller meals through the day, go ahead. If your body responds more to larger meals, feel free to do so. It is more important to make sure that you are not overeating your daily caloric limit than when you eat those meals.

If you partake in intermittent fasting, will you develop an eating disorder?

Intermittent fasting is not about developing an extreme eating pattern. It is a controlled pattern of eating during a certain time and not eating during another time. It is best matched up to your natural eating habits. The foods you eat are nutrient dense, so they are oftentimes healthier eating options that the foods you already partake in eating. Most people who do intermittent fasting do not develop an eating disorder. They actually become healthier from this lifestyle. However, if you have a history of the eating disorder or are concerned that you may develop one by beginning, consult your healthcare professional before beginning.

Does intermittent fasting or fasting cause you to overeat?

Interesting, when you begin intermittent fasting, the exact opposite tends to happen. Unless you are purposefully overeating, you will find that your appetite tends to change and you start to crave smaller portions. Remember, American portions are many times larger than what normal portions are across the world so the smaller portions would be considered normal portions worldwide.

Will I start to starve?

Gandhi was able to go on a hunger strike, only drinking water, and did not die. A few extended hours between meals is not going to cause you to starve or die. Our bodies normally have about a month's worth of stored fat available to us every day. So you will have a constant energy supply even if you intermittently fast.

Will I gain weight if I eat later in the day or late at night?

The best thing about intermittent fasting is that it fits into your lifestyle. You can choose to decide when to eat your meals. Of course, if you are eating lots of carbohydrates only, overeating and not eating vegetables or fruit with a late eating window, you may gain weight. The key is moderation and balance. If you are eating a normal portion at night, you should not see weight gain. Again, it depends on your body. Keep notes in your food journal to see how your body reacts to eating at a later window. If you are operating at a calorie deficit, you should be fine. The most important thing is not to overeat to avoid giving yourself a stomach ache and extra calories.

Will I lose a lot of muscle when I intermittent fast or fast?

When you eat, your body releases the nutrients you need steadily over time. Until you need to replenish nutrients from your next meal. Many people assume that fasting immediately causes muscle loss which is not the case at all. When you fast, remember you are still using the nutrients from your previous meal even if it was 16 to 20 hours ago. So realistically you will not lose muscle weight just by fasting in a certain window.

As you continue to learn about intermittent fasting, you will be surprised that it is actually quite healthy and has lots of benefits. Most of the misconceptions about intermittent fasting are resolved once you start practicing and see how the positive effect it has on your body.

Chapter 4: An Overview of Different Fasting Methods

In this chapter, we will take a look at things to be aware of when fasting and discuss fasting methods that are extended more than 24 hours. We will also add some hunger busting tips at the end of the chapter that will help you make it through any fasting time, no matter how short or long it is.

The great thing about intermittent fasting is that it is pretty flexible. Therefore you are able to adjust your fasting days according to what's best for you and your body. If you need to go out to eat with friends or family during a time that is your normal fasting time, you can just adjust your window to make sure you meet the fasting requirements for the day or you can make up the fasting time the next day. Another great thing about intermittent fasting is that you can drink water, black coffee or green or white tea during your fasting times to help you with your fasting periods. Weight loss is a welcome perk to intermittent fasting, but it is not the only perk. You may come to find that weight loss is just the cherry on top compared to other benefits of mental clarity and a lowered food bill.

For women, the best way to fast without throwing their hormones out of whack is to try to fast for 12 to 16 hours a day on two to three non-consecutive days. On the days that they fast, try to do light cardio or yoga. More intense workouts like strength or HIIT training can be done on the non-fasting days. Be sure to drink lots of liquids like tea, water, and coffee. If you are drinking tea and coffee, try not to put any sweetener or milk in it. You can also try to add a few amino acid supplements. If you feel comfortable, after 2 weeks, you can try to add another day of fasting. Not every woman is the same, and the results may vary per women. For women, it is important to go slowly and gradually to prevent adverse effects. Remember, you are not Superwoman or Superman, so take it slow to prevent hurting yourself and the people who care about you. Some people even like the form support groups of other minted fasters to encourage each other to keep going. This is especially helpful on the days that you want to work out.

Exercising with others who understand what you're going through and who are going through the same thing with you can be empowering, encouraging, and helpful as you tried to stay the intermittent fasting path. Other still like to hire a trainer that is familiar with intermittent fasting to make sure if they are tapping into the best workout that can leverage the intermittent fasting lifestyle. Whether you want to work out by yourself or with others on YouTube or in person or with a trainer, it is advisable that you continue to work out and do not give up exercise just because you are intermittent fasting. Exercising is still part of having a healthy lifestyle.

When you are intermittent fasting, it is important to pay attention to your body! Keep a food journal if you can. (You can buy one online or use a digital one.)As a matter of fact, it is all advisable. (More will be given on this later in the book.) A person should always be aware of the effects are having on their body. You will know that your body is not responding positively to intermittent fasting. If at any time, you notice these things, you should stop.

- **Insomnia** – If you are consistently staying up all night, and just can't sleep, then you need to stop intermittent fasting, so you look into the root cause of your insomnia further.

- **Extreme hunger to the point that you can't do anything else unless you are thinking about food.** – Intermittent fasting should be easy to do. Yes, at times, you will feel hunger. However, you should not be thinking about food so much that you are not able to function. There are a few tips you can use to alleviate your hunger pangs in Chapter 6 that can help you make it through your fasting windows. The truth of the matter once you get used to your fasting window, making it won't be an issue. The only concern you should have is if you can't make it through the intermittent fasting window and you cannot function AT ALL.

- **Weight gain, specifically in your mid-area**. – Unexpected weight gain, which is usually the opposite effect of intermittent fasting, should be cause for concern. If at any point, you notice unexpected weight gain, you should definitely reach out to your doctor.

- **Your period goes away or changes.** – For women, this is extremely important. If you notice any abnormal changes to your period while fasting, you may need to stop. Long term issues with your period could cause fertility issues so if you notice anything, speak out. If you think your ovulation is at risk or you feel like you are running into fertility issues, please, please, please reach out to your doctor.

- **You are especially stressed out.** – Intermittent fasting surprising helps people gain mental clarity. However, if you feel utterly and completely overwhelmed, it is okay to stop fasting, especially if you have low energy and can't concentrate. If you feel that your performance has declined tremendously because of fasting, do not be afraid to stop.

- **Skin and hair health** – If you notice that your skin's color looks off your hair seems thinner and brittle, this is a cause for concern. Any drastic changes with your hair and skin is an important indication that intermittent fasting isn't working.

- **Decreased bone density and muscle tone decreases.** – A change in your muscles or pain in your muscles can be a cause for concern. If you notice that your muscle tone has decreased or you feel pains doing your regular actions like walking the steps or getting in and out of cars, then you may want to reach out to your primary physician.
- **You begin to have a change in digestion.** – If at any point, you notice that you are having digestion issues that you were not having before, then intermittent fasting could be the cause. If there is extreme discomfort to where you cannot function, then reach out to your doctor. Some change in your digestion schedule is expected. However, if you notice something is way off, call the doctor.

- **You are always cold.** – Extreme coldness is another indication that you need to stop intermittent fasting. If you are colder than usual, and you have done everything you can to stay warm, but just can't stay warm. Then you need to reach out to your doctor.

The good news is that it is not all doom and gloom. However, there is a way to effectively practice intermittent fasting without falling into this vicious cycle, which is to begin fasting gradually. Do not begin all at once to prevent your body from going out of whack. More attention will be given to this in the next chapter. Ultimately, if you pay attention to your body, you will be able to tell if intermittent fasting is for you or not. Trust your body and listen carefully. It will let you know, so you do not have to be scared to try. Using the tips in this book will help you ease into the journey, so your body is not shell shocked.

When you fast, you need to also pay attention to the electrolytes that you are consuming. Electrolytes are the chemicals our bodies need to survive a fasted state. Electrolytes are already coming in our daily diet, but special attention should be given to them when you fast to make sure you are meeting your nutrient requirements in spite of fasting. Meeting the requirements are usually easy to do. As a matter of fact, most of us meet them every day without a hitch, but it is great to know what they are so you can be better prepared to handle intermittent fasting. After water, the most important ones are:

- **Calcium** – This is found in leafy greens like collard greens, spinach, kale, sardines, and dairy. You will know you have a calcium deficiency if you have muscle spasms or bone issues.

- **Potassium** – This electrolyte can be found in bananas, plain yogurt, and potato skins. If you have mental confusion, weakness of the muscles or paralysis of the muscles, you may have a deficiency.

- **Magnesium** – Found in pumpkin seeds, spinach, and halibut, it is important to have this electrolyte. Confusion, nausea or muscle cramps are an indicator that you may be deficient in this electrolyte.

- **Sodium** – This electrolyte is in soup, salt, tomato juice, dill pickles, and tomato sauce. You know you may need this electrolyte if you have a loss of appetite or muscle cramps or dizziness.

- **Chloride** – If you have an irregular heartbeat or changes in your pH, you may be experiencing a deficiency in these electrolytes. It is found in veggies like tomatoes, olives, lettuce and table salt.

The most important electrolytes to have while fasting are magnesium, potassium, and sodium. You should have about a teaspoon of salt a day and mix it with water; 2000 milligrams of potassium and at least 300 to 450 milligrams of magnesium. When you are eating, as long as you are eating foods rich in these electrolytes it can sustain you during the fasted stated. Eating healthy during your eating windows is just as important as not eating during your fasting periods. If at some point you feel comfortable with intermittent fasts, you can consider moving to extended fasts, starting with at least 24-hours.

Before you begin an extended fast, make sure you have consulted with a medical professional and are comfortable with your reasons for partaking upon the fast. Once you have this figured out, you will be able to move to preparing for the fast. You should know that extended fasting is perfectly safe and will cause you to reevaluate how you think of hunger. By the time you finish with your extended fast, you will no longer think of hunger as a negative. Daresay, you may think of it as a way to improve your mental health. And accept hunger for what it is – a brief moment that you can master. When you decide to do an extended fast, do not be afraid hunger, rather figure out ways to master it.

A Two-Week Fast Method

A two-weeks fasting protocol builds on all the other fasts. It's essentially water fast for 2 weeks. Before beginning this type of fast, you want to prepare. Before you begin, take the time to detox from unhealthy foods and habits like smoking and not getting enough sleep. The list of foods you will want to avoid consists of dairy, sugar, alcohol, eggs, fish, caffeinated drinks and meat. Try to eat raw foods every day for about a week before to make the longer fat easier to maintain.

After you have prepared, you can start the time to fast. You may be hungry but resist the urge to eat. The desire for hunger normally passes after three days. Stay hydrated to help you get through this stage. It's at this stage that people begin to think clearer and feel empowered. While staying hydrated, you also want to make sure you are taking your electrolytes. You can take them via supplements. You'll want to have magnesium, phosphate, calcium, potassium, and sodium. You will want to check with your preferred medical provider before embarking upon such a fast. A two-week can go fast quickly, and you can trigger fatal symports if you are not prepared properly. You may also experience extreme mood swings, so give your friends and family the heads up.

As you get deeper into the fast, you will start to feel fatigued, even dizziness, and sometimes blurred vision. Your breath can smell bad, and you may even get sick. This is your body's detox process. It shows that your body is responding well to the fast by getting rid of the toxins in your body. You may even experience some flu-like symptoms, like pains, aches, chills, and fevers. This is just your body's way of getting rid of the toxins by pushing them through your intestines, skins, lungs, nose, and stomach.

As some point, you will overcome the plateau. You will feel normal. You may even go back in forth between feeling sick and feeling normal. Again, this is your body responding positively to the fast. Stick it out if you can. If you notice any of the extreme symptoms from earlier in the book, that's when you want to reach out to your medical provider. If you can make it through a 2-week fast, you will feel amazed afterward.

For this type of fast, do not try to work out - just take it easy. Be thoughtful and meditate. To make it through the fast, you can stay in airy and bright rooms. When you fast, your body may give off an odor, so this will help it dissipate quicker. The bright room will improve your mood. Also, try to take in the sun for about 10 to 20 minutes daily before it gets too hot. To help with your breath, brush your tongue with activated charcoal powder. You can also scrub your skin with a dry brush and bathe multiple times a day to keep the odor at bay. To take the fast to another level, you can take two enemas daily during the first week and only once until the fast is over. One of the most important things is to surround yourself with people who care if you're going to make it. They will help you get through the tough times.

When it's time to break the fast, go extremely slow. The longer you go without food, the longer you need to spend slowly reintroducing the food back into your life. You can start with bone broth and then small meals. Don't try to eat everything at once. Go slowly. Most people prefer intermittent fasting, but a longer fast has immense health and spiritual or mental benefits. Ultimately, it's up to you to decide if an extended fast is best for you or not.

If you are still not sure if you can make it through the hunger pangs, here are some tips that can help. However, if you accept that hunger is a part of the fasting journey, you will have overcome one major hurdle. These tips can help you overcome and cope with hunger. They will be given as short-term strategies, long-term strategies, and a brief examination of what your craving and hunger can be telling you. By the time you finish reading, you'll be armed with all the necessary tools to bust hunger!

Short-Term Strategies

When you are hungry, you want to eat immediately. You do not have time to think about long-term solutions to your hunger. You need something fast and efficient to help you cope so you can make it through your fasting window. The strategies in this section will help you do just that. These strategies are intended to help you with the here and now. Make a note of the ones you think that are specifically helpful. Choose 1 to 3 methods to lean on as you begin to help you cope with your hunger. You can play around with the different methods until you figure out which ones are the best for you.

- **Eat a small snack.** If you do eat a snack, go for a snack that under 50 calories and low-fat. If you must snack, make sure you include them in your meal planning efforts.

- **Immediately distract yourself by playing a video game or another distraction to help you keep your mind off the hunger.** If video games are not your thing, try to get distracted by pleasurable activities, especially ones that burn calories like taking a jog around the neighborhood or calling and speaking with a friend.

- **Tap into the power of smell and smell something that smells like jasmine or vanilla**. Both are shown to help crave sugar cravings.

- **Take a nap.** Sometimes hunger is an indication of being tired, not being hungry. The next time you are hungry, take a quick nap and see if the hunger resides once you wake up. Worst case scenario, the nap will serve as a distraction from your hunger and you will wake up not feeling hungry at all.

- **When that hunger pang hits, floss and brush your teeth.** You can even put a minty lip chap on with the hopes of the mint stopping you from getting too hungry. You can also pop a strong mint like an Altoid. The mint flavor should encourage you not to eat and mess up the freshness of your breath.

- **Take a deep breath or do a few quick yoga poses** to help clear your mind, and stop your cravings.

- When your next craving hits, **take the time to do for tea.** Make a fancy tea time with a cup of hot tea. You can also do a nice cup of ginger tea as ginger has been shown to help stop cravings. Avoid sugary pastries and sweeteners during this tea time. You can also try fancy infused water, with mint, pomegranate, basil or cucumber or your favorite fruits instead. If tea or water isn't your thing, just do coffee instead. Remember, to limit the sweeteners and try to drink everything without creamer or sugar.

- Using **acupuncture techniques** is another way to try and curb your hunger. Tap your forehead for 30 seconds or try pinching your earlobes and nose.

- Another popular remedy to curbing your hunger is to **chew gum, especially after lunchtime**. Chewing gum can help you make it to your next eating window. Be sure to go for the sugarless variety. If you notice that you have any stomach issues after chewing gum for long periods of time, select a different, hunger coping mechanism.

- **Use your imagination and let yourself give in mentally.** Imagine yourself eating whatever you want as a way to satisfy your hunger.

- **Think about how eating your craving will affect you in the future**. Will eating bring you closer or further away from your goals. Thinking of the long-term effects of not sticking to your fast may prevent you from eating during the fasted state.

- **Just ignore the hunger pains**. They typically last for 15 minutes. They come in bursts. If you can hold off for 15 minutes, you should be home free.

- **Take a spoonful of apple cider vinegar after you eat or even before a meal**. If you take it after you eat, the apple cider will help you make it through your fasted window. If you take the apple cider vinegar before you eat, it can help curb your appetite before you eat. If you take a spoonful while you are hungry, it can help you make it through your intermittent fasting window.

- **Worst case scenario: just give in and eat**. Eat a very small portion, chew slowly and enjoy it. If you really give in, try to forgive yourself. We aren't always perfect, and sometimes we have to eat. However, try to go without eating for as long as you can before you give in. Try not to make it a habit.

Long-Term Strategies

The strategies in this section aim to help you create habits that will help you long term on your intermittent fasting journey. Depending on your personality and your budget, these strategies can be easy or more difficult to implement. These strategies are ones that you should try once you have figured out that you are committed to being an intermittent faster. Even if you are not committed after you give it a test drive, some of these methods will still help you monitor your food intake. Ideally, your goal should be to incorporate these tips and let them become a habit to help to make intermittent fasting for your easier.

- **Try to coordinate your intermittent fasting with your schedule you are already following**. Keep in mind that after about five hours, unless you are sleeping overnight, your blood sugar levels drop and you begin to crave food. If you can craft your fasting and eating windows with this concept in mind, it will be easier with you to deal with your hunger.

- **Try to avoid purchasing high fructose corn syrup**, because it is an additive. If you eat something with high fructose corn syrup in it, you will tend to want more of it. If you want some, it can cause you to want more. Other names high fructose syrup go by includes: fructose, maize syrup, glucose syrup, fructose or glucose syrup, tapioca syrup, fruit fructose, crystalline fructose or HFCS. Anytime you see one of these names your intermittent fasting antennae should be up and you should try and avoid that food.

- Next, **try to avoid eating refined sugar** which is often found in white sugar, white flour, or white pasta. Try to replace it with natural sweeteners, nut flours, or whole grain pasta or forgo these ingredients all together.

- **Purchase blue plates for your home.** Blue plates are shown to help prevent cravings. This may be a little pricey so do not be afraid to check second-hand stores for this item. Also, try using smaller plates that will help limit your portions sizes. You can also use bigger forks to help you become fuller in a shorter amount of time.

- **Try to get more sleep.** If we do not get enough sleep, that's when you can begin trying to compensate with unhealthy eating choices. Sleeping is crucial to achieve a healthy lifestyle. This is one area where you do not want to skimp on. Give yourself seven to eight hours a night and watch the difference it will have in your life. Your mood will improve, your weight will improve, and your productivity will improve. Sleeping is underrated. Give it a try and watch how it affects your life.

- **Create a list of items to do that calms you, makes you happy or that you enjoy.** Try to let them be things that do not involve eating. Try to create 25 things and pick one the next time you are hungry pick one from the list.

- **Are you an emotional eater?** If so, try to get to the root cause of why you are eating when you are emotional. Remember that journal you were supposed to keep from earlier? Be sure to note any trends of when you are eating if you are bored, stressed, sad, or mad, then adjust your behavior accordingly. Be mindful of what you are eating so you do not eat because you are bored or stressed.

- Just like hunting for high fructose syrup or refined sugars, **get into the habit of reading food labels**. You'll want to pay special attention to the serving size. This will help you not if you are overeating or not. Also, saturated fats and sodium are other categories that you want to pay attention to and choose foods that are high in fiber. When you add more fiber to your meal, it helps you make it through your fasting periods easier. You'll also want to pay special attention to the vitamins and minerals in the food to make sure it is full of good food for you.

- **Make the lights brighter when you eat your meals.** This is an interesting tip and may be on the pricey side if you need to buy a few new or brighter bulbs. Bright lights raise the awareness of what you are eating; whereas, dim lights tend to lower your inhibitions. This means when the lights are low, you tend to pig out. Keep those lights bright, so you do not overeat and effectively ruin your intermittent fasting eating window.

- Another quick way to help you watch what you eat and prevent you from pigging out during your window is to **have a soup or salad as an appetizer first**. You can also have a cup of water first. This tip can fill you up with good nutrients and help you not to overeat.

- Although it sounds counterintuitive, **you will want to eat the same foods every day.** This helps your body to adjust easier and helps make meal planning easier to make sure you are getting the proper nutrients and calories that you need. If you are a person who believes that spice is the variety of life, do not be afraid to try new things after at least eating a set schedule for a few days to see how your body reacts. The best to back your diet is with foods that are bulky but low in calories like whole grains, beans, fruits, and vegetables.

Whether you are interested in adding short-term or long-term strategies to your life, both of these categories can help you make it when you feel like your stomach is going to fall through your back. Again, pick one to two strategies to start with, and note them in your food journal. You will be able to track and see which methods work the best for you and which ones are keepers and which ones you need to replace. The next section will deal with a different aspect of your hunger. It will focus on your cravings and how to tell if your cravings are telling you something or not. What our cravings tell us can be especially helpful to our meal planning and overall health.

A 24-Hour Fast Method

One of the easiest ways to break into a longer fasting period is to start with a 24-hour fast. A 24 hour fast is great for giving your physical body a reset. It helps reset your system for issues related to your appetite, gut, and energy. When you begin this fast, you want to still go through your regular routine. When your fasting for 24 hours or longer, try to stay away from food so you won't be tempted and try to keep your mind clear from thinking about food. Remember, anyone can fast up to three days without any medical supervision. If you are doing an alternate day fast or a 5:2 fast, you can slowly transition to going to one full day of not eating.

The night before you begin your fast is very important, so make sure that you are eating a balanced meal. Get up and start your day like normal. You can even start off with tea or water or coffee. And go through your regular activities. By the time you finish, you will notice that your 24 hours have gone by quickly. Once it's time to break the fast, don't just eat a huge meal. Slowly ease into the meal, so you don't get sick. Start off by drinking a nice warm glass of lemon water that will prepare your stomach for the coming meal. Wait thirty minutes and then have a low carb snack. Wait another thirty minutes and then eat a nice, well-balanced meal. Also, don't overdo the meal. After any fast, do not eat everything you see to avoid gaining unnecessary weight. Control your urges so you can get the most out of your fast. Also, don't be alarmed if you have to go to the bathroom more after you fast. It's your body's natural reaction to your higher metabolism that may occur after a fast. You can take a probiotic before eating to try and regulate your urge.

A 36-Hour Fast Method

A 36-hour fast is extremely helpful for those who have type 2 diabetes due to their higher insulin resistance compared to those with type 1 diabetes. For this type of fast, it is recommended that a person does it 2-3 times a week for those with type 2 diabetes. People who don't have diabetes will also benefit from this fast. One of the easiest ways to do it is to have dinner around 6 or 7 pm on Day 1. On Day 2, you wouldn't eat any meals, only drink fluids with no calories added. Then you wouldn't eat until 6 or 7 am on the third day. It may feel weird at first, but this type of fast is definitely doable.

A 42-Hour Fast Method

A 42-hour fast builds on the 36-hour fast. You would still have dinner around 6 pm on Day 1. On Day 2, you wouldn't eat any meals, only drink fluids with no calories added. Then you wouldn't eat until noon on the third day. An easy way to transition into a 42-hour fast is to get into the habit of having your first meal around noon-time. To start this habit, in the morning, you would wake up and have a cup of coffee or water. If you get into the habit of having your first meal around noon, your body won't feel as hungry when you first wake up.

It is important to remember that when you are doing a longer fast, you don't want to restrict your calories. Eat normal sized meals, but don't overdo it. You may think that you will want to eat everything in sight once you finish your fast, but you may realize that your appetite goes down. So eating until you are full does not result in a huge feast like expected.

What Your Desire are Telling You!

We all get hungry, but some of us never pay attention to what we are craving for at the moment. In order to survive, our bodies want certain nutrients, vitamins, and minerals to sustain us. Sometimes, we just want good old' water. The following section details what our cravings could be telling us. When you are writing in your food journal, pay special attention to what you are craving and what days. Noting the time and if you are craving these foods after any certain activities will also provide insight into what you are craving.

Keeping careful track of your cravings can help you figure out what you are craving and in some cases why. It will help you take your combatting hunger to another level. By focusing on what your hunger is telling you, you are making sure you are meeting your dietary needs as well as possibly catching any disturbing signals that your body may be telling you. Sometimes our bodies give similar signals for certain cravings, but the best thing to do if you are not sure what to do is to drink water. It typically helps with cravings and satiates hunger. Do not underestimate the power of paying attention to what your body is telling you. Listen and watch your body reward you for it.

Sweet foods

Just like salty foods, sugar craving is a good indicator that you need to drink more water. This craving is also related to your caffeine intake and your sleeping schedule. A sugar craving can also be your body's way to stay energized. So if you down lots of caffeine and barely are getting any sweets, try to get some sleep and lay off the caffeine as well. Another way to help ease this craving is to incorporate more naturally sweet fruits and vegetables into your diet, like carrots, sweet potatoes, beets, apples or vegetables into your diet. Instead of sugar, you can try natural sweeteners such as agave or maple syrup instead of sugary snacks and drinks. Honey is touted as helping you feel full longer so do not overlook this favorite sweetener or many. If you are always craving something sweet, try something sour to kill the craving. Sour foods also help improve your digestive system. Lastly, incorporating more protein in your diet can also help you overcome the sugary diet as your body will be sustained and you do not have to rely on sugar to pick your body up.

Salty foods

This is a good indicator that you need to drink more water. Our body responds to being dehydrated by craving salty foods. This is a common craving people have. If you have it, let an 8-ounce cup of water sooth it. Along with water, increase your intake of calcium, magnesium, and zinc. Make sure that you are not experiencing exhaustion, extreme weight loss or a change in the color of your skin. This could point to a larger health issue if you are craving salt all the time. To encourage you to drink more water, you can purchase a cool water bottle or personalized one that you already have to your liking. This will give a special touch to your water drinking. If you are a person who despises water, see if you can start with sugarless sparkling water or invest in sparkling water machine to make your own sparkling water at home. You can also consider infusing the water with different fruits to give it a taste. There are no ways around not drinking water. You just have to find a way to cope with drinking it that is to your liking.

Soda

Craving a carbonated, sugary soda suggests that you may have a calcium deficiency. Increase your calcium intake to help with this craving. You can find calcium in leafy green vegetables if you are vegan and other plant-based sources so do not feel that you only can find calcium in dairy. If you are craving the carbonation so you can burp, try sparkling water or club soda with fruit infused in it to see if it will give you that same field. Sparkling water is a much healthier option than soda, and it gives you some of the same joys of burping that soda does.

French Fries and Potato Chips

A craving such as this means that you need to eat more healthy fats found in oily fish like salmon, sardines or nut. If this is a persistent craving, you should also consider adding more fiber, magnesium and chromium food that is found in foods like chard, celery, spinach, apricots, apples, and bananas. If you just can't seem to rid yourself of the potato chip or French fry craving, create your own healthier options from sweet potatoes or white potatoes. You can also thinly sliced vegetables and create your own crunchy vegetables by roasting them with a little extra virgin olive oil in the stove. These are healthier alternatives, and you may become addicted to them just like you are to French fries and chips.

Chocolate, Cheese, and Dairy Products

If you are craving chocolate or cheese, you may need to pick up your mood. Chocolate and cheese are known as comfort foods and rightfully so since they release feel-good chemicals to improve your mood. If you notice that you are having these types of cravings, look for ways to boost your mood like taking a quick jog or doing a few quick stretches at your desk. If you are still struggling with chocolate and dairy cravings after trying to improve, you can consider looking into vegan options or eliminating it from your diet altogether. Ridding themselves of dairy has helped a lot of people with their health journey, and if you do that on your intermittent fasting path, you may be surprised at the results.

Ice or Red Meat

This could point to an iron deficiency. If you have low iron, increase your protein intake or even eat more red meat. If you are vegan or vegetarian, see about increasing your intake with beats of plant-based sources or protein. Make sure this craving is not coupled with any drastic skin or hair changes, as well. Iron is an important aspect of a healthy lifestyle, so don't overlook this craving if you have it.

Any other desires

Drink more water to try to help the craving. Also, note if you can tell any weird other things happening with your body such as extreme weight loss or weird mood swings or any other dramatic changes. Some food cravings can point to pregnancy if you are a woman or other health issues for men and women. Always err on the side of caution. If you feel like something weird is going on, trust your instincts. Health Care Providers are there for a reason. Don't be afraid to reach out to them.

If you are eating a well-balanced diet, then your craving issues should be easier to manage and control. Not just a well-balanced diet, but drinking a lot of water is helpful, too. The next section will focus on more tips to help you get through your non-eating periods and answers any questions you may have.

Chapter 5: Fasting Recipes

Breakfast Recipes

Egg, Toast, and Turkey Bacon Cups

This recipe takes preparation time of 10 minutes, the cooking time of 20 minutes, and makes 12 cups.

One serving contains:

- 10 grams Protein
- 11 grams Carbohydrates
- 8.5 grams Total fat

What to use:

- Eggs (12)
- Turkey Bacon Slices (12 cooked 75% of the way)
- Whole Wheat or Gluten Free Bread (12 slices)

What to do:

1. Preheat the oven to 375 degrees. Before you start assembling the steps, go ahead and have your turkey bacon slices cooked at least 75%. The turkey bacon will finish cooking while in the cut.

2. After you get the turkey bacon settled, go ahead and remove the crust from each side of the bread slices, and smash each piece of bread with a baking pin. Try to get it as flat as possible.

3. Then cut a circle into the bread. Once the circle is cut, cut the circle diagonally.

4. Spray a muffin tin well and place the diagonal halves in the muffin space. Be sure not to have any space showing on the bottom.

5. Then cut the turkey bacon in half and place each one in an individual cup on each side of the muffin tin. You can have at least one half of the turkey bacon higher than the side. Once the bread and the turkey bacon are arranged, you can bring out the eggs.

6. Break the eggs into each muffin space. You do not have to scramble them.

7. Bake for at least 20 minutes or until the egg is to your preference.

Simple Chia Pudding

This recipe takes about 6 hours and 5 minutes to prepare and makes 4 servings.

The serving size is 0.5 g. It contains:
- 6.9 grams Protein
- 3 grams Sugar
- 9.5 grams Fiber
- 16.3 grams Carbohydrates
- 23 milligrams Sodium
- 4.3 grams of Saturated Fats
- 10.3 grams Fat

What to use:
- Extract (Vanilla) (1 teaspoon)
- Agave (1-2 tablespoons)
- Dairy-free milk (1.5 cups)
- Seeds - Chia (0.5 c)

What to do:
1. First, combine the maple syrup, vanilla extract, chia seeds, and dairy-free milk in a bowl. Then whisk the ingredients very well to mix them all together.

2. Refrigerate the ingredients overnight or for at least 6 hours in the bowl (preferably overnight), so the chia pudding is thick and creamy. If the chia pudding is not thick and creamy, you can add more chia seeds. Then put it back into the refrigerator, and keep it in the refrigerator for about another hour or so until the pudding is firm. You can garnish it with fruit or almonds or nuts of your choice.

Quinoa and Cinnamon Breakfast Bowl

This recipe takes preparation time of 5 minutes, the cooking time of 15 minutes, and creates 2 portions.

A serving contains:
- 14 grams Protein
- 15 grams Sugar
- 8 grams of Fiber
- 94 grams Carbohydrates
- 6 grams Total fat

What to use:

- Fresh fruit of your choice (2 c)
- Maple syrup (2 tbsp)
- Cacao nibs (2 tbsp)
- Salt (to taste)
- Extract (Vanilla) (0.5 tsp)
- Cinnamon (to taste)
- Milk (Non-dairy or dairy) (1 c)
- Water (Filtered or Purified) (1 c)
- Uncooked quinoa (1 c)

What to do

1. When you begin, rinse the quinoa well and drain the excess water off. Place the quinoa to the side.
2. Then put the quinoa, water, and almond milk in a saucepan and boil it.
3. When the quinoa and the mixture starts boiling, reduce it to a simmer and season with the salt and taste of vanilla.
4. Turn off the heat when the liquid is gone. When it is finished, fluff the quinoa and top with the fruit, maple syrup, and cacao. Add more liquid to thin.

Sweet Potato Kale Hash

This recipe takes 10 minutes of getting it ready, 35 minutes to cook it all, and makes 2 servings.

A serving contains:

- 15.7 grams Protein
- 9 grams Sugar
- 6.8 grams Fiber
- 37.3 grams Carbohydrates
- 911 milligrams Sodium
- 12.8 grams of Saturated Fats
- 18.8 grams Total fat

What to use:

- Kale bundle (1 large one)
- Ground turmeric (0.125 teaspoons)
- Fresh parsley (2 tablespoons)
- Red onion (1)
- Salt and pepper (0.5 teaspoons each)
- Coconut sugar (1 teaspoon)
- Tandoori Masala spice (3.25 teaspoon)
- Melted coconut oil (2 tablespoons)
- Sweet potatoes (2 small ones)
- Extra-firm tofu (8 oz package)

What to do:

1. Pre-heat your oven to 400 degrees Fahrenheit. Before you make the tofu, you want to get it as dry as possible so it

will crisp up nicely and be extra crispy.

2. To dry out the tofu, take the tofu out of the package and put the tofu in a clean towel. Then put a skillet or pot on the towel that is on top of the tofu so it can squeeze out the extra moisture. If the towel becomes soaking wet while following this step, you can replace it with another clean towel.

3. While the tofu is frying, chop the sweet potatoes into small cubes and season them. Next, slice the onions and season them as well. Then, combine the onions and potatoes onto a lightly greased baking pan.

4. Bake the potatoes and onions for 25 to 35 minutes and flip them one time while cooking so both sides can be nice and brown.

5. You will know they are finished cooking when the onions are caramelized and brown and the sweet potatoes are tender. Remove the potatoes and onions from the oven. Put them in another bowl so they won't keep cooking on the tray, and set them to the side.

6. While the potatoes and onions are cooling, put the dried out tofu in a bowl and scramble it well with two forks. The tofu should be scrambled into small pieces, and they will look like scrambled eggs somewhat.

7. Then, in your large skillet, heat the cooking oil, add all your spices, and sauté your tofu for 5 minutes. You want

to get the tofu as brown and dry as possible without burning it. Set the finished tofu aside.

In the same pan, put a little extra oil and sauté your kale, followed by adding your tofu back in. Divide the kale, sweet potatoes, onion, and tofu into bowls equally and serve.

8. You can serve with hummus or a hot sauce.

Fantastic Breakfast Salad

This recipe takes preparation time of 5 minutes, the cooking time of 15 minutes, and it makes a single portion.

A serving contains:

- 29 g Total fat
- 3 g Sugar
- 17 g Protein
- 13 g Carbohydrates
- 7 g Fiber

What to use:

- Salt (to taste)
- Avocado (0.3 of the avocado and make it sliced)
- Roasted cauliflower (0.5 c)
- Baby greens of kale, spinach or your favorite (2-3 c)
- Chopped red onion (0.25 c)
- Eggs or egg substitute (1 to 3)
- Cooking oil of your choice (2 tsp)

What to do:

1. Sauté the onions until they are soft in the extra-virgin olive oil.

2. Then add in the roasted cauliflower and greens to the skillet. Sprinkle with a pinch of salt. Put the mixture into a bowl.

3. Then add more oil to the skillet, and make the two eggs how you like it. Once the eggs are ready, put them on top of the salad.

4. You can add a little hot sauce and sprinkle with ginger to take it to another level.

Lunch Recipes

Grilled Salmon and Grapefruit Salad with Olive Oil

This recipe takes preparation time of 15 minutes, the cooking time of 10 minutes and creates 4 portions.

A serving contains:

- 21.2 grams Protein
- 2.5 grams Fiber
- 2.1 g Saturated Fat
- 35.8 grams Carbohydrates
- 493 milligrams Sodium
- 2.1 g Polyunsaturated Fat
- 5.3 grams MSG
- 10 g Total fat

What to use:

- Grapefruit sections (1 24 oz jar)
- Mixed baby salad greens (8 cups)
- Cooking spray
- Large onion (1 cut into 0.5 inch thick slices)
- Ground black pepper (0.25 tsp)
- Salt (.05 tsp)
- Extra-virgin olive oil

What to do:

1. Get your grill ready. Spread it liberally with cooking spray so the food will not stick to it.

2. Season your salmon, coat with cooking oil or spray and onion slices. Place the onions and fish on the grill rack coated with cooking spray.

3. Then grill until the onion is tender and the fish is flaky.

4. Place two cups of salad greens on four serving plates. Then put the onions into chunks, grapefruit sections, fish, and onion.

5. Then drizzle with extra-virgin olive oil.

Black Bean Salsa Burgers with Potato Circles

This recipe has a preparation time of 5 minutes, a cooking time of 8 minutes and creates 4 portions.

A serving contains:

- 14 grams Protein
- 5 grams Sugar
- 9 grams of Fiber
- 74 grams Carbohydrates
- 669 milligrams Potassium
- 318 milligrams Sodium
- 3 grams MSG
- 1 gram Polyunsaturated Fat
- 1 gram Saturated Fat
- 6 grams Total fat

4What to use:

For the Potato Circles

- Paprika (0.4 of a teaspoon)
- Oregano (Dried) (0.75 of a teaspoon)
- Parsley (Dried) (0.75 of a teaspoon)
- Garlic Powder (0.5 teaspoons)
- Baking Potatoes (2 large ones sliced thinly)

For the Burgers

- Extra-virgin olive Oil (1 tablespoon)
- Your favorite salsa (0.25 cup and 2 tablespoons)
- Brown Rice Flour (0.5 of a cup)
- Old Fashion Oats (0.5 of a cup)
- Black beans (a 15 oz cup)
- Lettuce wraps (optional)

What to do:

For the Potato Circles

1. Start your oven to 450 degrees.
2. Mix the potatoes up with the spices, and put them on a baking sheet that has aluminum foil. You can also choose to spray the baking sheet liberally with extra virgin olive instead.
3. Roast them for about 20-30 minutes, tossing them

halfway through.

For the Burgers

1. Mash the black beans and all the ingredients except the extra-virgin olive oil into one bowl. If the mixture seems too wet, you can mix in more flour. If your mixture seems too dry, add 1 tablespoon of salsa, one tablespoon at a time.
2. Separate the mixture into four equal sections and flatten them into patties.
3. Refrigerate them for 20 minutes.
4. Then put oil into a skillet and fry each patty until crispy.
5. Eat using your favorite toppings, including your favorite bun. For a healthier option, you can eat the patties in a lettuce wrap. You can also choose to add a low-fat or non-dairy cheese option to the burger as your 'cheese.'

Simple Lentil Soup

This recipe takes preparation time of 15 minutes, the cooking time of 20 minutes, and creates 7 cups.

The serving size is 1 cup, and it contains:

- 8 grams Protein
- 4 grams Sugar

- 8 grams of Fiber
- 24 grams Carbohydrates
- 250 milligrams Sodium

- 11 grams of Saturated fat

What to use:

- Fresh lime juice (2 tsp)
- Baby spinach (1 5 oz pack)
- Pepper (Cayenne) (to taste)
- Pepper and salt (according to taste)
- Low salt vegetable broth (3.5 c)
- Uncooked red lentils (0.75 c rinsed and cooked)
- Coconut milk (1 can, 15 oz)
- Tomatoes (Diced) (1 can, 15 oz)
- Ground cardamom (0.25 tsp)
- Cinnamon (0.5 tsp)
- Cumin (Ground) (1.5 tsp)
- Turmeric (Ground) (2 tsp)
- Garlic Cloves (Minced) (2 large cloves)
- Onion (Diced) (2 c)
- Cooking oil (1.5 tbsp)

What to do:

1. Sauté the minced garlic cloves and diced onions within the large pot in the cooking oil for about 4 to 6 minutes over medium heat until the onion is soft. Put in the salt and fry it until it is fragrant.

2. Add ground cardamom, cinnamon, turmeric, and cumin and stir until combined well. Continue to cook for about one more minute until it smells nice.

3. Then add a full can of coconut milk and a can of diced tomatoes, including the juices. You can put in the cayenne pepper to taste if you feel like it.

4. Stir all the ingredients together until it is combined. Then increase heat until it reaches a low boil.

5. When it begins to boil, turn down the heat and let it cook until the lentils are tender.

6. Turn it off and add the spinach until it wilts. Add in the lime juice then decide if you want to add more salt and pepper.

7. You can serve with toasted bread of your choice, a leafy salad or vegetables. This recipe also holds up well in the refrigerator so you can prepare a huge batch and freeze it for later.

Chilled Lemon Zucchini Noodles

This recipe takes 25 minutes to prepare, and it makes 4 servings.

A serving contains:

- 19 grams Fat
- 8 grams Carbs
- 2 grams Protein
- 5 grams of Sugars

What to use:

- Salt and pepper (to taste)
- Lemon (1 zested and juiced)
- Mustard (Dijon) (0.5 teaspoons)
- Powder (Garlic) (0.5 tsp)
- Cooking oil (of your choice) (0.3 c)
- Zucchini (3 medium ones cut into noodles)
- Radishes (1 bunch thinly sliced)
- Thyme (1 tbsp chopped)
- Cauliflower florets (optional)
- Broccoli florets (optional)
- Low-fat or dairy-free cheese option (optional)

What to do:

1. Combine the lemon zest and juice, powder garlic, and mustard in a small container. Whisk them all together.

2. Slowly add in cooking oil of your choice. Again, whisk it all and combine. Use salt and pepper to season it according to how your taste buds like it. When it is mixed well, you can go ahead and put it to the side to prepare the rest of the ingredients.

3. Wash the zucchini, and you can peel it or decide not to. Once it is peeled or not, you can go ahead and cut them with a Zoodler.

4. When the noodles are ready, in a large bowl, toss the zucchini noodles and radishes.

5. You can add in your dressing sitting in your bowl to the side and toss until the veggies are well coated.

6. Garnish with fresh thyme and serve. A modification to this recipe is you can add as many vegetables as you like. You can consider adding broccoli or cauliflower florets. You could even add chopped pepper as well. To take it to another level, you can choose to add a low-fat or dairy-free cheese option, too.

Cauliflower Nachos with Turkey Meat

This recipe takes preparation time of 15 minutes, the cooking time of 25 minutes, and creates 4 portions.

A serving contains:

- 27 g Protein
- 29 g Fat Total
- 14 g Carbohydrates
- 6 g Fiber
- 5 g Sugar

What to use:

- Fresh Cilantro (2 tbsp)
- Avocado (0.5 medium avocado)
- Red onion (sliced 0.3 cups)
- Tomatoes (diced 0.75 cups)
- Cheddar cheese (1 cup shredded)
- Turkey sausage (1 pound)
- Taco seasoning (1 tsp)
- Avocado oil (0.25 cup)
- Cauliflower (1 large head)
- Salsa (optional)
- Guacamole (optional)

What to do:

1. Start your oven up to 425 degrees. Put grease on your baking sheet and oil it well. Cut the cauliflower into florets and slice them as thinly as possible to make chips. Toss the cauliflower chips with the taco seasoning and avocado oil.

2. Roast them for about 20 minutes on the sheet as a single layer until browned and crispy on the edges.

3. While the cauliflower is roasting, go ahead and cook the turkey sausage for about 10-12 minutes until you do not see any pink.

4. When the cauliflower is finished roasting, flip them over and place the cooked meat over the top of it.

5. Add cheese, red onion, and tomatoes. Then let it in the heat till the cheese melts nicely.

6. You can garnish it with cilantro and avocado. You can add your favorite salsa and guacamole mix or chop a few tomatoes and avocado to make a tomato and avocado salad.

Dinner Recipes

Green Vegetable Juice with Apple

This recipe takes 5 minutes to prepare, and it makes 1 serving.

A serving contains:

- 1 gram Protein
- 8 grams Sugar
- 3 grams Fiber
- 13 grams Carbohydrates
- 191 milligrams Potassium
- 10 milligrams Sodium

What to use:

- A sweet Apple (1 peeled and cored)
- Fresh parsley (a large handful)
- Kale leaf (1 large one)
- Romaine leaves (3)
- Cucumber (half of a medium sized one)
- Raspberries, cherries or blueberries (optional)
- Chia seeds or hemp seeds (optional)
- Protein powder (optional)

What to do:

1. Wash all of your ingredients well and juice them all until smooth.
2. Drink as soon as you finish.
3. You can modify this by adding green or white tea, apple juice, aloe vera juice, low-fat yogurt, Greek yogurt or water to thin it out.
4. You can also garnish with nuts or seeds or extra fruit. For an extra dose of protein, add a scoop of your favorite protein powder to the mix.

Pineapple Rice with Grilled Steak

This recipe requires 15 minutes of preparation time, the cooking time of 20 minutes and creates 4 portions.

A serving contains:

- 345 milligrams Sodium
- 31 g of Protein
- 52 milligrams Calcium
- 44 g of Carbohydrates
- 6 grams Sugar
- 2.8 grams of Saturated fat
- 3 grams Monosaturated fat
- 0.4 grams Polyunsaturated fat
- 4 grams of Fiber

- 10.3 grams Fat

What to use:
- Black pepper (0.5 tsp)
- Salt (0.9 tsp)
- Precooked Brown Rice (8.8-oz)
- Soy sauce (light sodium) (0.25 c)
- Beef tenderloin fillets (4 (4-oz))
- Cooking spray
- Pineapple slices (1 (8-oz) can, drained)
- Green onions (6 pieces)

What to do:
1. Make sure your meat is well washed, and the fat is trimmed before you begin the recipe.
2. In a large plastic bag, mix together the low-salt, soy sauce, pepper, and beef. Let the beef marinate and stay at room temperature for about 7 minutes. Turn the bag every now and then, so the marinade mixes with the beef well. The more the marinade gets in the meat, the more it will be flavorful.
3. While the steak marinates, heat the grilling pan sprayed with cooking oil. Put the green onions and pineapples in the grill and cook it until they are well-charred. Once they are cool, cut the onions and pineapples into bite-sized

pieces.

4. Cook the pre-cooked rice according to the directions. Then add the pineapples and the green onions to the rice.

5. Once the rice is done, then cook the beef in the grill pan until it is done. You can grill it for 3 minutes on each side until it is done or cooked to how you like it. When it is finished cooking, you can serve the beef with the pineapple rice.

Lamb Chops in Orange-Vinegar Sauce

These instructions require a cooking time of 15 minutes, a cooking time of 10 minutes, and create 8 portions.

A serving contains:

- 12.1 grams of Total Fat
- 25 grams Protein
- 2 grams Carbohydrates
- 5.4 grams Monosaturated fat
- 582 milligrams Sodium
- 0.6 grams of Polyunsaturated fat
- 2 grams Sugar
- 4.6 grams of Saturated fat

What to use:

- Olive oil (tsp 4)
- Grated orange rind (tsp 2)
- Orange juice (tbsp 1)
- Cooking spray
- Lamb rib chops (8 (4-oz) fat trimmed)
- Salt (according to your taste)
- Black pepper (according to your taste)
- Balsamic vinegar (3 tbsp)

What to do:

1. Before you begin, wash your lamb well. Make sure that your workspace has your raw meat separate from your vegetables and other food to prevent cross-contamination.

2. Combine a tablespoon of orange juice, olive oil, and orange rinds in one plastic bag large enough for the marinade. Marinate the lamb well for at least 10 minutes at room temperature.

3. Remove and then season well with seasoning.

4. Warm up the grill and coat it with a liberal amount of cooking spray. Then cook the lamb chops on both sides for about 2 minutes until it is done to your preference.

5. Then take the lamb chops off and place the balsamic vinegar in a small skillet. Cook until the balsamic vinegar is syrupy (maybe about 3 minutes). Put a tablespoon of

extra-virgin olive oil. Then drizzle the vinegar and the mixture over the lamb chops.

6. This would be awesome with corn on the cob or even a small leafy salad, spread with the same vinaigrette sauce.

Cucumber Chickpea Salad

These instructions require a preparation time of 10 minutes and create 4 servings.

A serving contains:

- 13 grams Protein
- 6 grams Sugar
- 9 grams of Fiber
- 30 grams Carbohydrates
- 272 milligrams Potassium
- 608 milligrams Sodium
- 9 grams MSG
- 11 grams Polyunsaturated Fat
- 3 grams of Saturated Fat
- 25 grams Total fat

What to use:

Tahini Dressing

- Water (0.25 c to thin)

- Salt (0.23 teaspoon)
- Garlic clove (1 that's minced)
- Lemon zest (1 lemon)
- Juice (1/2 small lemon)
- Balsamic Vinegar (3 tablespoons)
- Tahini (cup = 0.25)

Salad

- Parsley (Chopped and fresh 0.25 cup)
- Red onion (cup =0.25, diced)
- Chickpeas (a 15 oz can, rinsed and drained)
- Cherry tomatoes (1 pint, halved)
- English cucumber (1, chopped)

What to do:

1. Mix all the salad ingredients very well in one bowl.
2. Mix the dressing ingredients, except water, in a separate bowl.
3. Add a tablespoon of water to the dressing until it is as thin or thick as you would like. If you want to thicken it up, add more tahini to the mix.
4. Then add the dressing and stir everything again.
5. Eat or keep it in the refrigerator until it is ready to be eaten. You can serve on toasted bread of your choice or with crackers. You can also dip vegetables into it and

enjoy it as a snack.

Lentil Mushroom Tacos

These instructions require 5 minutes of preparation time, the cooking time of 20 minutes and create 6 servings.

A serving contains:

- 14 grams Protein
- 3 grams Sugar
- 10 grams Fiber
- 40 grams Carbohydrates
- 936 milligrams Potassium
- 450 milligrams Sodium
- 1 gram Total fat

What to use:

- Water (0.5 cups)
- Cayenne Pepper (a teaspoon of 0.5)
- Cumin (a teaspoon of 0.5)
- Smoke paprika (0.5 teaspoons)
- Garlic powder (a teaspoon of 0.5)
- Salt (according to your taste)
- Chili powder (tablespoon =1)
- Baby Bella mushrooms (a 16 oz package)

- Lentils (2 cups)
- Toasted bread (optional)
- Steamed vegetables (optional)
- Lettuce wraps for the tortilla (optional)
- Low-fat or non-dairy cheese (optional)

What to do:

1. Before you begin, have your lentils already prepared.
2. Then wash the mushrooms and chop them well. Then sauté the mushrooms in a skillet until they are soft. You do not have to add any oil as mushrooms give out a lot of moisture. If you feel the mushrooms are sticking, you can add a little water.
3. Then add the cooked lentils, water, and seasonings, mixing them well.
4. Simmer the mixture until everything is heated through.
5. You can serve in a lettuce tortilla for a healthier option. You can also serve with a side of mixed vegetables or sprinkle dairy or low-fat cheese across the top when it finished cooking.

Snacks Recipes

Bakeless Kiwi Cheesecake

These instructions require at least 25 minutes of preparation time, a freeze time of at least 3 hours, and make 6 servings.

A serving contains:

- 24 g of Carbohydrates
- 3 g of Fiber
- 16 g of Sugar
- 2 g of Protein
- 8 g of Total fat

What to use:

For the topping

- Blueberries (optional)
- Raspberries (optional)
- Fresh mint
- SunGold Kiwis (2)
- Green Kiwi (1)

For the cheesecake layer

- Green kiwi (1)
- Mint leaves (1)
- Agave or rice syrup (tbsp 2)
- Lime juice (2 tbsp)
- Milk (Coconut or non-dairy) (0.75 full-fat)
- Cashews (2 c, soaked

for at least 4-6 hours   or at least overnight)

For the crust
- Dates (1 c)
- Almonds (1 c)

What to do:

1. Pulse almonds until nicely crushed. Then add the dates and blend them again until a sticky mixture forms. Then press it into a 7-inch springform pan, and put in into the freezer.
2. Next, make the cheesecake layer by draining the cashews. Combine the cashews with the coconut milk, lime juice and agave in a blender until it becomes creamy and smooth.
3. Then put about 75% of the cashew mixture evenly onto the base layer and put it back into the freezer.
4. Leave the rest of it in the blender, and add one kiwi, then the fresh mint leaves. Blend it all together up until the mixture is smooth and light green. Put it on top of the already freezing layers, and put it back in the freezer for 2-3 hours.
5. Take it out about 20-30 minutes before it is ready to serve. You can drizzle it with agave or rice syrup and then top it with the fruit.

6. This is a very popular dessert. It also pairs well with a hot drink like a green tea or infused lemon water.

Twice-Baked Vegan Sweet Potato Skins

The instructions require a preparation time of 15 minutes, a cooking time of 15 minutes, and create 4 portions.

A serving contains:
- 34 g of Carbohydrates
- 4 g of Protein
- 6 g of Fiber
- 544 mg of Potassium
- 310 mg of Sodium
- 6 g of Sugar

What to use:
Toppings (Optional)
- Hot sauce
- Chopped cilantro
- Your favorite salsa
- A low-fat or non-dairy cheese sauce
- Avocado
- Sliced green onions
- Sautéed peppers

Potatoes

- Corn (0.25 c, can be thawed frozen corn or fresh)
- Black beans (0.25, drained and rinsed off)
- Hot sauce (2-4 tbsp)
- Dairy-free yogurt (0.25 c)
- Salt (a smidge)
- Extra-virgin olive oil (drizzle for baking)
- Sweet potatoes (4, 2.5 by 4-inch ones)

What to do:

1. Preheat your oven to 350 degrees Fahrenheit.
2. Wash the potatoes. Then rub them with broth or oil to get the salt to stick.
3. Bake the sweet potatoes in your oven for at least 45 minutes.
4. Once tender, remove them from the oven. Then let them cool for a little bit before slicing them. Then when they are cool, slick them in half.
5. Scoop out the insides. Be sure to leave a small edge on the inside.
6. Once they are scooped out, put the potatoes, inside side down, to crisp the outside of the potatoes.
7. Then mix the potato insides with the yogurt and hot sauce. Add the corn and beans. Mix everything very well together. Take the skins out the oven and put the mixture

on the inside of them.

8. Bake it all again for 10-15 minutes.

9. Then you can top it with whatever toppings you would like.

Grilled Chicken and Pineapple Sandwiches

These instructions require a preparation time of 6 minutes, a cooking time of 10 minutes, and it makes 4 servings.

A serving contains:

- 0.9 g of Saturated Fat
- 4 grams Total Fat
- 30.5 g of Carbohydrates
- 1 gram of Monosaturated Fat
- 43.4 g of Protein
- 1.4 g of Polyunsaturated Fat
- 608 mg of Sodium
- 4.1 g of Fiber

What to use:

- Cooking spray
- Boneless and skinless chicken breasts (4 6-oz halves)
- Salt (0.5 tsp)
- Light mayonnaise
- Black pepper (0.25 tsp)
- Juice of 2 fresh limes
- Pineapple slices (4, 0.5-inch thick)
- Whole wheat hamburger buns (4 toasted or lettuce wraps)
- Basil (4 large leaves)

What to do:

1. Prepare grill and spray a lot of cooking spray liberally.

2. Season the chicken well and grill them. Every now and then, brush the chicken with lime juice.

3. Then grill the slices of pineapple and assemble your sandwich by adding chicken, grilled pineapple slice, and a basil leaf to each sandwich.

4. Spread mayonnaise on bottom halves of buns, if desired.

5. A good modification is to add a lettuce bun.

Fresh Orange Sorbet

This recipe takes 15 minutes to prepare and 2 hours and 8 minutes to cook, and it makes 12 servings.

A serving contains:

- 0.4 grams Protein
- 23.1 grams Carbohydrates
- 0.2 grams Fiber
- 1-milligram Sodium
- 5 milligrams Calcium

What to use:

- Oranges (10 medium ones)
- Water (2.5 c)
- Fresh lemon juice (0.33 c)
- Grated orange rind
- Sugar (1 c)
- Mint sprigs (optional)
- Rosemary (optional)

What to do:

1. Remove the rind and white pit from an orange very carefully. Then cut the orange rind into longwise thin

strips.

2. Segment the peeled oranges to half sections, then squeeze the juice until it equals 0.33 cup.

3. Combine the sugar and water to a pan and boil, then add the orange rind strips to pan.

4. Turn the heat down and cook it slowly for 5 minutes. Drain the mixture, so no pulp is left. Only save the liquid and discard solids. Cool it.

5. Next, add orange and lemon juice to the sugar liquid, and stir.

6. You can then pour the totality of the liquid mixture into an ice-cream freezer for the tabletop and freeze the orange sorbet as written by the manufacturer.

7. Spoon sorbet into a freezer-safe container; cover and freeze for 1 hour or until firm. You can top it with the grated rind and mint sprigs if desired. You can also add a sprig of rosemary as a garnish.

Sweet Power Balls

These instructions require a preparation time of 45 minutes, and it makes 25 servings.

The serving size is 1 ball; it contains:

- 19 milligrams calcium
- 72 milligrams potassium
- 13 milligrams sodium
- .6 milligrams iron
- 1 gram of fiber
- 1.4 grams carbohydrates
- .7 grams protein

What to use:

- Shredded unsweetened coconut (.75 c)
- Honey (.5 c)
- Room temperature sunflower butter (.3 c)
- Sesame seeds (.25 c)
- Semisweet chocolate chips (.3 c)
- Diced dried plums (.5 c)
- Puffed rice (1 c)
- Puffed millet (.5 c)

What to do:

1. Mix the puffed millet and rice together with dried plums, sesame seeds, and chocolate chips.

2. Mix in the honey and sunflower buttons and then cover and refrigerate in the bowl for a total of 30 minutes.

3. Put the shredded coconut in a separate bowl. Then using a tablespoon, scoop the mixture and form it into a 2.5 cm ball. Shape the ball with your hands and roll the balls in the shredded coconut and put in a container.

4. A good modification would be to use dark chocolate chips.

And there you have it! You have five recipes that you can use for breakfast, lunch, dinner, or snacks that can help you begin your intermittent or fasting journey. Good luck!

Conclusion

Thanks for making it through to the end of *"Intermittent Fasting: The Complete Guide For Weight Loss, Burn Fat Through Meal Plan, Healing your Body for a Healthy Lifestyle."* Let's hope it was informative and able to provide you with all of the tools you need to achieve your goals whatever they may be.

Fasting is not new to humankind. From the beginning of time to modern time, the benefits of fasting have been lauded by philosophers and health practitioners alike. Some of the earliest indications of the benefits of fasting were to deal with sickness. Researchers today have shown that intermittent fasting is indeed healthy, and it has many benefits that can help you live a long and healthy life. For Americans who are dealing with unhealthy lifestyles, intermittent fasting may just be the solution that they are looking for. The journey to intermittent fasting is an easy one to start, but maintaining it can be difficult. Whether you are afraid of not being able to make it through your fat and window or just scared that your body will go haywire once you begin, you can overcome them all if you make a slow and gradual approach to intermittent fasting. If you feel incredibly concerned, reach out to your doctor. So, what do you have to lose? This book has given you everything that you need to know, and I hope it has alleviated any fears that you may have about intermittent fasting.

We have attempted to give you an overview of what intermittent fasting is, how it benefits your lifestyle, and why you should be doing it. The following chapters gave you an overview of what intermittent fasting is, what fasting is all about, and how you can get started today.

In Chapter One, we talked about fasting (including its brief overview) and the benefits it can have on your life. In Chapter Two, practical tips on how to fast were given and also the steps to help you begin. We explored the different versions of extended fasting and some advice to curb your hunger while fasting in the Third Chapter. Chapter Four answers all the questions you may have about fasting, and, lastly, Chapter Five gives you a bountiful of recipes to entice you on this "one of a kind" diet regimen. All the chapters demonstrate that fasting is doable, feasible, and a reasonable lifestyle choice for people who want to be healthy.

I hope that you do not delay in starting your intermittent fasting lifestyle. The quicker you begin, the faster you can experience improved health results, let alone in overall health goals. So, how about you? What's holding you back? There should be no more excuses.

The next step is to make a real commitment to start intermittent fasting. Decide what method you are going to use. Which window will fit best into your life as it is now? Would it be 5:3, 16:8, 12:12, or eat a day and skip a day? Whichever one it is, pick that method. Go throw away all your junk food, make a meal plan, and get started! I wish you all the best! I cannot wait to see and hear all your wonderful stories! Soon, you will join the ends of people who know the power of intermittent fasting, and you will revel in the healthier lifestyle that you now have, thanks to the many benefits of an intermittent fasting lifestyle. When you look back at the time you were not intermittent fasting, you will be able to laugh and smile knowing that you are now doing what you thought at one time was impossible. You will find yourself grinning by the fact that there is sweetness in the stomach emptiness that you are now privy to enjoying.

The *"Intermittent Fasting: The Complete Guide For Weight Loss, Burn Fat Through Meal Plan, Healing your Body for a Healthy Lifestyle"* can be used as a resource anytime you need encouragement or to double-check any question about intermittent fasting you may have. We'll end with the words of Plato, "I fast for greater physical and mental efficiency." Maybe you are like Plato. Perhaps you want to fast for the mental and physical benefits for yourself. Maybe you are trying to be an example for your friends and family. Whatever your reason for fasting is, you may run into snags but don't let them stop you. Get started today!

Finally, if you found this book useful in any way, a review on Amazon is always appreciated!

Description

What if I tell you all about a fantastic way to help you live longer, lose weight, and that is super easy to do? If you are struggling with weight loss and have no idea what to do to get it under control, this book can help. If you do not like to exercise that much, but still need to lose weight, this book is for you. If you want a lifestyle that our ancient ancestors used, then this book is for you! When you read, *"Intermittent Fasting: The Complete Guide For Weight Loss, Burn Fat Through Meal Plan, Healing your Body for a Healthy Lifestyle,"* you will learn all the ways intermittent fasting, and fasting in general, can help you in your life!

Besides losing weight, *"Intermittent Fasting: The Complete Guide For Weight Loss, Burn Fat Through Meal Plan, Healing your Body for a Healthy Lifestyle"* will also explain all the benefits of intermittent fasting and fasting which includes:

- A practical, lesser-known way to control Type 2 Diabetes,
- A simple way to improve your appearance,
- Useful tips to start fasting and help you manage your hunger,
- An overview of all the intermittent fasting options you can

choose from

- Answers to all the burning questions you may have surrounding intermittent fasting, and
- Easy, money-saving recipes to help you start planning your meals for maximum nutritional benefits, as well as a beautiful, simple way to improve the hormones in your body (which allows your cells to run more efficiently and healthily),
- And more!

Fasting's power is in the ease of how simple it is. Whether you have never been concerned about your health and hate exercise or if you are a super-duper health nut, anyone can do it. Once you start intermittent fasting and see how easy it is, you will not want to quit! Pick up *"Intermittent Fasting: The Complete Guide For Weight Loss, Burn Fat Through Meal Plan, Healing your Body for a Healthy Lifestyle"* so you can start intermittent fasting today!

www.ingramcontent.com/pod-product-compliance
Lightning Source LLC
Chambersburg PA
CBHW051350280526
45784CB00007B/2890